UNSTOPPABLE:

Zap Fatigue
& Zoom Ahead

Hugo Tschudin

LEGAL INFORMATION

Publisher. First published as an ebook by Hugo Tschudin (htschudin@tschudin.com / EnergizingLifePublishers (www.EnergizingLife.com).

Disclaimer: Individuals and medical or other professional theories differ and keep changing. The author is not a *medical* doctor (but a research specialist and magna-cum-laude Doctor of Law of the University of Basel, Switzerland). So the information presented here is no substitute for the *personal* attention of competent, *up-to-date* medical, nutritional, psychological and other professional service providers. Any application is at the reader's discretion, and is his or her sole responsibility.

Library of Congress Cataloging-In-Publication Data:
Tschudin, Hugo.
UNSTOPPABLE: *Zap Fatigue & Zoom Ahead* / by Hugo Tschudin

(1) Lifestyle (2) Fatigue (3) Overcome Fatigue (3) Energy (4) Increase Energy (5) Energize Life (6) Success

Library of Congress Number: 2013918711

HUGO ("The Pep Doctor") TSCHUDIN

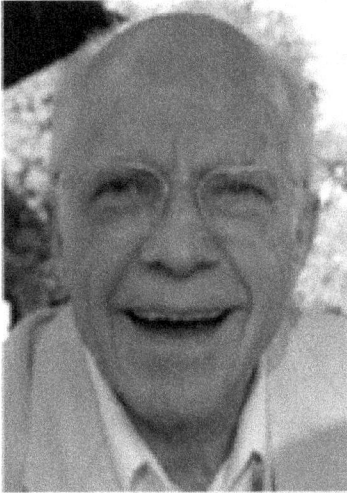

I'm one of those fortunate individuals who somehow managed to turn their most frustrating weakness into their greatest strength. MY WEAKNESS—the one that almost ruined my life—WAS FATIGUE.

UNFORTUNATELY, my perennial weariness was slowly but steadily increasing. Already as a pre-teen, I had great difficulties getting up in the morning. My health was fragile, and my teachers thought I couldn't stand the rigors of academic studies.

FORTUNATELY, I didn't listen. I gave it my best, graduated from the University of Basel (Switzerland) with a magna-cum-laude Doctor-of-Law degree, and became a legal research assistant.

UNFORTUNATELY, my fatigue continued to get worse when —upon immigrating in the United States in 1958—I worked first as a trainee and then as an executive in three Manhattan companies, and later started my own management research company (with up to 12 employees).

FORTUNATELY (yes, fortunately!) my "fatigation" became unbearable ... so bad, in fact, that I finally took corrective action when I was already 75 years old.

I EXPERIMENTED with extensive lifestyle changes, and tapped into the knowledge of psychologists, psychiatrists, nutritionists, physiologists, conventional and holistic physicians, sleep researchers, motivational consultants, NLP practitioners, stage and medical hypnotists, biographers of great achievers, etc., to learn all I could about fatigue, energy and related subjects.

MAJOR RESULT NO. 1: I came up with a checklist of the most effective energizing strategies I had uncovered. Subsequently, I used it to prepare a highly concentrated, time-saving booklet entitled <u>Wake Up to Abundant Energy: 113 Ways to Make It Easy to "Rise and Shine"</u>.

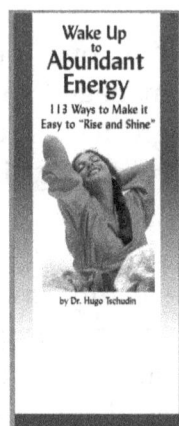

MAJOR RESULT NO. 2: I put my know-how into action and turned my life around. I now fall asleep in less than ten minutes, sleep *very* well, wake up refreshed, alert and cheerfully in the morning, and get up promptly and easily.

AT 84 YEARS OF AGE, *I have more early-morning and daytime "oomph" than I had in my twenties.*

MY PASSION AND MISSION: Now that the bane of my life morphed into my greatest blessing, I help my readers and "mentees" to also: (1) conquer early-morning exhaustion and misery, and (2) increase daytime energy and improve their overall performance and their quality of life.

NOW IT'S YOUR TURN! With much more energy from the very beginning of every day, you'll be far better equipped to meet the challenges *and opportunities* coming your way during your waking hours.

YOU WILL DISCOVER that "everything" will become much easier and much more gratifying for you.

USE THIS BOOK as your *Wake-Up Call, Workbook and Guide* to: more stamina, endurance and accomplishments ... greater success and prosperity ... more options, fun and happiness ... and above all more zest for life!

Let it help you to become UNSTOPPABLE ... to ZAP FATIGUE AND MOVE AHEAD!

TABLE OF CONTENTS

PART I

WHAT'S IN THIS BOOK FOR YOU

A. Yes, you can choose to wake up with lots of energy every day (including Mondays!)

a. You don't have to take fatigue lying down

Dear Reader:

Do you get that *feeling of utter gloom and exhaustion* when the alarm shatters the stillness of the night?

You know what I mean. It's that sense of exhaustion and powerlessness that weighs a ton on your body and mind.

When you wake up, you're supposed to be energized, but you are *not—au contraire!*

If this is your problem, you're not alone. Ongoing scientific investigations point up that *fatigue is a serious and growing threat* to the quality of our lives.

Having enough energy to cope with the relentless stress thrust upon us is an ever-present challenge in our high-strung 24/7 society. It's also the root-cause of many of today's most devastating chronic illnesses.

Major studies do, indeed, paint a rather disturbing picture. According to the National Sleep Foundation, 49 percent of Americans wake up tired *at least* two days a week. More recent investigations indicate that our problems are getting worse. Only 8.9 percent of us wake up well rested. A shocking 38 percent begin their waking hours downright exhausted.

> *Instead of beginning our waking*
> *hours with all the energy we need*
> *to get up immediately and take on*
> *the challenges and opportunities*
> *that lie ahead in good cheer, we're*
> *already washed out before we*
> *even lift a finger!*

For many of us, our work is a perennial "drag." Sadly, we don't even get much satisfaction and joy out of our "own time" afterwards and on weekends.

The low level of energy we start out with every day impairs everything:
• our relationships,
• our work and success
• our self respect, and
• the quality of our lives.

This is deplorable and *TOTALLY UNNECESSARY!*

b. Perennial fatigue isn't "fate"

If you're "energy-challenged," *please don't assume that fatigue is your "fate"*—not even if (like me, Hugo Tschudin) you've had a "fatigue problem" for decades and are by now convinced that you're stuck with it for life (just as I was until a few years ago).

Fortunately, research also brings to light with growing persuasiveness that ...

> *We don't have to take fatigue lying down. We can take corrective action. WE CAN FIGHT BACK!*

So, if you awake dejected, drained and downcast ... if it's a tough battle for you to get out of bed and confront the challenges that lie ahead ... and if you're tired a lot also during the day: take heart!

> *You can finally zap fatigue and zoom ahead!*

There's a body of *helpful know-how within your easy reach*. You'll probably find more of the most powerful methods to fight "Early-Onset Fatigue Syndrome" (a new term of mine for lexicographers and drug manufacturers to ponder) in this book than in any other single source of information.

The strategies you'll find straight ahead are based on real-life, down-to-earth *experimentation* (mine) as well as *scientific investigations* spanning the spectrum from psychology to "self help," from motivation to autosuggestion, and from pharmacology to holistic medicine (to mention just a few for the time being).

> *With this books, it's now up to you to tap into the wealth of*

information that you will need,
and to make smart choices that are
geared to your personal needs and
aspirations.

As I found out through trial and error as well as lots of interdisciplinary research, *we can "energize" ourselves to an astonishing degree*—even at an advanced age.

To illustrate, here is a true "story"—*mine*.

This is not merely a narrative of how "lucky me" (Hugo Tschudin) solved a distressing "fatigue problem."

It also contains important eye-openers for *whoever* wishes to get rid of the shackles of *untimely* fatigue (not the fatigue resulting from a healthful workout at the gym).

c. How I got rid of "Early-Onset Fatigue Syndrome" (and you can, too)

I was once in the same boat you may still be in now.

I had difficulties getting up already in my primary-school days in my home town (Basel, Switzerland). I was a some-what frail kid, and my mother had to call me again and again to have me emerge from the bed covers.

Rising became gradually even more troublesome in my adult years, especially in my sixties and seventies. (I'm eighty-four years old now.)

Every morning, it took me at least
half an hour to climb on my feet.
Getting ready was "just awful."

I stumbled around like a zombie, and often could not find some of the clothes I wanted to wear even though I had laid them out the night before.

I staggered around, bumped into furniture, forgot what I wanted to do next, what to take along to work, and so on.

I usually managed to hide my misery from my family by moving out of their way. Or I camouflaged how I felt with a phony smile. But I could not hide the truth from myself, and that was the worst of it.

Here I was, a grown-up man. Early-on, while I was still a student in Switzerland, I had become president of the Efficiency Club of Basel, an organization of over 1,000 businessmen aspiring to high achievements.

And after having immigrated into the United States, and having been employed in responsible positions in three companies in Manhattan, I had established a management consulting firm with up to twelve employees.

I had been striving for greater
performance for decades.

Yet I could still hardly get moving in the morning. I idled in bed although there was so much work to be done. It was shameful. My "laziness" was "awful," and getting worse.

I was not a failure. But I should have been more successful considering the sacrifices my hard-working parents in Switzerland had made to give me a first-rate education.

> *During all these years, I was tired a lot,*
> *and this undoubtedly held me back in*
> *my career. I was also not very happy.*

It took me more and more of an effort to get up.

My "character weakness" got to be so distasteful to me that I finally decided to carry out whatever research would be necessary to take corrective action.

d. Sporadic remedial efforts led nowhere

When I made the decision to investigate, I was already 75 years old. That's when I "woke up" and started experimenting.

I tried numerous new lifestyle approaches, usually inspired by magazine and newspaper articles which I happened to come across—articles on subjects such as "How to Select Mattresses for More Restful Sleep" or "The Seven Secrets to Increasing Your Energy."

My most delightful experiment involved an *alcoholic "nightcap."* I started sipping a Swiss chocolate-cherry liqueur. It did, indeed, make me "nod off" sooner. But when its sedative effect vanished (usually sometime after midnight), I invariably woke up, and then tossed and turned in bed for most of the rest of the night. So this did, regrettably, not work.

Trying to go to bed earlier and earlier to "gain more energy" did not help me either.

On the contrary, it elongated the time it took to fall asleep. And the longer it took, the more worried I became that I could not do my work properly on the following day.

I did not get much sleep for several nights in a row, and was afraid of losing my sanity.

I popped *sleeping pills* and had great difficulties weaning myself of this pernicious practice.

More harmless but equally disappointing was my experience with a "Sunrise-Simulation Alarm Clock." It illuminated the bedroom with increasing intensity before the actual alarm sounded off.

But the effect of the intensifying light wasn't strong enough to make getting up any easier.

I also tried *other approaches* including various:
• dinner hours,
• bedroom temperature settings,
• linen, blanket and pillow types,
• bedtime rituals (relaxation, breathing, mind-control, etc.),
• herbal and other sleep aids, and so on.

Some changes were beneficial at least for a while. But nothing was quite good enough.

Then, one day, I came upon a learned article about *"psychological fixations."* I lost it but remember that, according to its author, fixations are hard to get rid of because they're *anchored in the depths of our subconscious minds.*

But we can overcome them with appropriate know-how and sufficient determination, he wrote. We can, he asserted, even overcompensate their negative effects, thus turning our weaknesses into strengths, and defeats into triumphs.

e. Systematic wide-angle research finally did the trick

The notion of fixations (hang-ups) was not new to me, of course. But now I had a fancy term for it, and realized for the first time that casually arrived-at conclusions need to be questioned and sometimes replaced with carefully considered new concepts.

This insight—coupled with my worsening *"Early*-Onset Fatigue Syndrome"—caused me to decide to *initiate a veritable in-depth research project* to find the right solution to my problem.

Using the investigative skills I had acquired in my diverse previous occupations (law, new-product development, market research and executive selection), I did something unusual:

> *Rather than just "sticking to my knitting,"*
> *or tapping into one single knowledge base*
> *(such as medicine or psychology), I began to*
> *use a wide-angled multidisciplinary approach.*

To accomplish this, I combed through the know-how not only of sleep specialists but also of:

- psychologists,
- psychiatrists,
- physiologists,
- nutritionists,
- medical practitioners,
- pharmacologists,
- sports coaches,
- motivational consultants
- NLP practitioners,
- hypnotists,
- biographers of great achievers, and
- other professionals.

To access their expertise, I studied uncounted books, research reports and abstracts, "white papers," professional magazines, articles, websites, blogs, etc.

f. Proof is in the pudding

I tested the experts' recommendations (using myself as the guinea pig), and arranged the ones that "did the trick" for me in *checklist* form for my own easy future reference.

Later, I used the checklist to prepare a booklet entitled <u>Wake Up to Abundant Energy: 113 Ways to Make It Easy to "Rise and Shine"</u>.

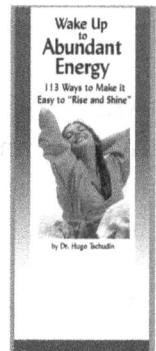

Ever since I put these strategies to good use in my own life—those I had developed myself and the ones I had gleaned from leading specialists—I haven't had any more sleep- and fatigue-related problems.

Defying some of the negative stereotypes of "seniors," I usually:
- fall asleep in less than ten minutes,
- sleep *very* well,
- wake up refreshed, alert and cheerfully,
- get up promptly and easily, and
- *keep my energy at a high level throughout the work day.*

I don't *always* feel great. I don't *always* follow my own advice. But overall, I'm doing extremely well.

> *After having learned to "zap fatigue,"*
> *I now have—at the age of 84 years—*
> *more early-morning and daytime*
> *energy than I had in my twenties.*

g. It's your turn!

After having benefited from my investigations, I now help my readers and "mentees" (the counterparts of "mentors") to master the same methods that helped me beyond my fondest hopes to:

(1) conquer my early-morning exhaustion and misery, and
(2) increase my daytime vitality and productivity, and
(3) improve the overall quality of my life.

> *With more energy, "everything" becomes*
> *so much easier and more pleasant!*

We wake up fully rested, begin and continue our days with a positive mindset, and can enjoy life much more fully.

May this book serve as a *wake-up call and guide* for my readers, their families and friends, who—like me until a short time ago —dislike or even hate to get up, and would love to wake up with an abundance of energy and stamina.

From the time I made my life-changing decision to look for solutions to my "energy problem," it took me almost three years to reach my ambitious "energy goal."

> *You can attain the same gratifying*
> *results in a fraction of this time*
> *because you're beginning your*
> *"upturn" with the know-how that*
> *only extensive experimentation*
> *and research could bring.*

The difference this book can make in *your* life is likely to *exceed your expectations* by a huge margin. The reasons are spelled out in the following section.

B. Why starting your days with abundant energy is a "must" for making the most out of your life

a. Waking up—a blessing or a bane for you?

The way we start your days—whether we loathe it or love it—largely determines the quality of our lives.

It controls far more than just how we experience the *first minutes* of every day.

Usually, it preordains the course of our affairs *throughout* the day. (In addition, its influence often extends far into the future, as we will see later.)

This is why we often say of a normally well-balanced person that he "got up on the wrong side of the bed," or "got off on the wrong foot" on days when he is late ... or in a bad mood ... or can't seem to get his act together ... or gets into arguments ... or makes more mistakes than usual as the day unfolds.

These terms imply that he was tired and miserable upon waking up and *therefore* had a "bad day." The energy with which we are endowed upon waking up does, indeed, matter. It makes a *huge* difference in our waking hours:

(1) Persons who wake up fully energized:

> For them, mornings are "just wonderful." They can get on their feet right away and with practically no effort. Within a minute or two of waking up, they are moving around at

full speed, with their minds in gear. Because they want to make the most of their time, they don't dilly-dally and mope around. Rather, they proceed to their activities promptly and in a perfectly positive frame of mind.

(2) Persons who wake up tired:

Their "life scripts" are different. They hate the sound of their alarms, start out drained, drowsy and ill-tempered. They waste precious time to gather the strength they need to get up. And when they're finally on their feet, they often feel somewhat dizzy. They may need a super-sized mug of coffee to clear out their "brain fog."

For the unfortunate individuals in this second category, early morning is an unpleasant daily occurrence at best.

For some it's a horror. One blogger lamented that he hates getting up so much that he also hates going to bed the night before. Getting up is so abhorrent to him, he wrote, that it "mars my entire life."

But this is unfortunately not the end of the tribulations.

b. Misery drags us down and usually gets worse

Furthermore, the early-morning distress of "energy-challenged" individuals is not limited to the first hour or two of wakefulness. It usually continues in multiple ways throughout the day.

(a) Misery inertia:

> The fatigue with which we wake up
> rarely stops when we're out of our beds,
> groomed, dressed, fed, and on our way.
> Rather, it has "staying power."

Just notice the *worn-out faces* around you when you commute to work, and upon arrival.

Many of your colleagues *must rely too much on coffee or soft drinks,* or on donuts, cookies, chocolate, candy or other high-calorie snacks, to get the *energy jolts* they need to buckle down to work. And they need additional "fixes" whenever their caffeine- and sugar-induced energy spikes wear off.

If they remain stressed out throughout the day, they may even be *too tired to fall asleep* soon enough at bedtime.

Their fatigue is likely to continue on the following day, and perhaps even longer, until they decide—like I some time ago —to take life-changing corrective action.

(b) Misery escalation:

In addition to dragging on, fatigue and the resulting distress usually also *intensify.*

On their way to work, energy-challenged commuters often *get even more "sick and tired"*—for instance when other drivers swerve toward them or force their way in ahead of them. (Incidentally, most traffic accidents occur between 6:00 and 9:00 a.m.—when many of us are still not totally awake).

*Upon arrival at their workplaces,
lack of "oomph" will often make it
difficult for them to tackle their real
work. Their growing backlog and
fatigue may take an increasingly
heavy mental toll.*

Poor performance and its consequences (such as disapproval or criticism from customers, colleagues and superiors, and the resulting damage to their self-esteem and earnings) often exacerbate their weariness.

(c) Rebound effects:

In a fatigued state, they're rarely in complete control of themselves.

They overreact and tend to be unfriendly, grouchy, ill-tempered, overly critical, and in danger of becoming unbearably negative and cynical.

Their *victims* feel unappreciated and treated unfairly. They *may withhold their cooperation and support.* They may also *retaliate* by opposing and *slandering* them openly or behind their backs.

*Such ricochet effects can hit them and
drag them down right away. Or they
may harm them in weeks, months or
years to come.*

(d) Business success impediments:

Continuing fatigue will prevent many of us more than anything else from developing our full potential in the world of work.

It diminishes our endurance, concentration, and our reasoning- and problem-solving powers.

> *Other damaging consequences*
> *of low energy include absenteeism,*
> *lagging productivity, frequent*
> *mistakes, poor work quality, low*
> *self-confidence, and difficulties*
> *holding on to good positions.*

(e) Career and earnings limitations:

Succeeding in demanding settings—such as in positions held by executives and traveling sales professionals—is next to impossible for the "energy-challenged."

> *Clawing one's way to the top of*
> *the ladder, and fending off fierce*
> *competition, are not for the faint-*
> *of-heart, the surly, the weak and*
> *the perennially fatigued.*

Those who make it to the top are usually the most energetic, dynamic and upbeat individuals.

They're also the ones who *earn the highest compensation.*

(f) Spare-time flops and doldrums:

Coming home exhausted, and taking their frustrations out on family members, or escaping to the wasteland of mindless TV viewing, are inauspicious ways to get their spare time underway.

> *Fatigue mars not only the time that's*
> *available for family and friends, but also*
> *for fun, hobbies, recreation, sports,*
> *advancing their education, and other*
> *pursuits that make life particularly*
> *worthwhile.*

(g) Health problems:

The consequences of the fatigue, frustrations and stress that begin already when it's time to get up have health consequences that may be *more insidious* than all of the above repercussions *combined.*

They trigger the fight-and-flight response. When this happens, the sympathetic nervous system (the one acting without conscious thought) causes the adrenal glands to *inundate the blood stream with adrenaline, cortisol and other stress hormones.*

If the stress persists long enough, it will cause *increasingly serious illness* that can affect every part of the body:

• *Circulatory System:* heart disease (including heart attacks), hypertension, arteriosclerosis (incl. circulation problems in arms and legs, such as varicose veins), and aneurisms (bulges in artery walls),

- *Digestive Tract:* gastritis, stomach ulcers and cancer, ulcerative colitis and colon cancer, hemorrhoids,
- *Reproductive Organs:* menstrual disorders, vaginal infections, impotence, premature ejaculation, prostatitis, prostate cancer,
- *Brain:* strokes, depression, chronic insomnia, personality changes,
- *Muscles:* neck, shoulder and other types of musculoskeletal pain,
- *Skin and Hair:* eczema, psoriasis, excessive hair loss, and some types of baldness.

This list of health problems caused by continuing fatigue and stress is far from complete. But the above organ systems are particularly vulnerable to the ravages of the "daily grind."

In addition, stress can *aggravate virtually every other illness.*

C. The many expected and unexpected ways this book will benefit and enrich you

a. What's at stake for you?

The above list of consequences of low personal energy is eye-opening and disturbing.

Obviously, sluggishness, lethargy, gloom, listlessness and other manifestations of fatigue cramp our lifestyle. *They define our personalities negatively and limit our potential.*

Conversely, high energy enlarges our potential, possibilities and power, and multiplies our chances of growing, developing, achieving, flourishing and finding happiness.

Reducing this to a common denominator, we can say:

> *"As is your energy, so goes*
> *your life."*

But all this is abstract and somewhat impersonal. For a more complete appreciation of *what's at stake for you,* you may want to give some thought to the following questions.

Do I want to reach the following goals:
☐ Wake up full of energy and in a positive frame of mind every morning?
☐ Rise within seconds or minutes, thus putting an end to what may be my single biggest daily waste of time ?

☐ Get on my feet with no trouble at all—without struggling, and with virtually no effort?

☐ Have all the energy I need from the beginning to the end of my waking hours, so I can cope easily with the challenges and opportunities that are bound to come my way?

☐ Avoid being ensnarled by "brain fog?"

☐ Get ready for the day's activities cheerfully and efficiently (without spilling coffee, forgetting to take important belongings with me, etc.)?

☐ Look and feel better—*a lot* better—all the time?

☐ Navigate the trip to my work place with equanimity and imperturbability (not letting the "small stuff" affect my good mood)?

☐ Arrive at my destination early, with a can-do spirit and a smile on my face?

☐ Cheer up stressed and tired colleagues, customers and others?

☐ Tackle tough tasks right away rather than dilly-dallying?

☐ Do my work cheerfully, efficiently and well—without becoming *dependent* on coffee, donuts, sugary and other fattening fare to cope with fatigue and depression?

☐ Have enough "pep" left over after work for enjoyable evenings with family, friends, hobbies or sports, and whatever else I value highly in my life?

b. What makes this book especially beneficial?

There's probably no shortage of books and articles offering energy- and mood-enhancing know-how ... but:

> *What may put this book in a class*
> *by itself is its main focus on the*
> *beginning of the day.*

This is *the time when we have the biggest need for energy*—the time of transition from sleep to wakefulness.

It also determines more than any other time how the *entire* day will turn out for us (such as whether we are likely to reach our goals, cope well with challenges, experience joy and satisfaction, etc.).

In addition, how we feel when we gain consciousness is the *best marker of the health of our minds and bodies.*

The book is equally unique in other ways:

(a) It's the farthest-reaching handbook on making getting up easy.

It draws not just on one or two areas of expertise (such as sleep physiology or neurochemistry), but cuts across many categories of knowledge.

(b) It focuses on 69 powerful strategies. While not every one of them is of equal value to everybody, there's safety in this high number because there's plenty to choose from.

The strategies are broad-based and were picked with great care. Obviously, I alone am responsible for their selection.

(c) It gives readers the practical know-how they are likely to need. But it leaves out academic or other baggage that doesn't contribute to the understanding of real-world problems and their solutions.

(d) It explains why the strategies are generally effective (unless, of course, the reasons are obvious).

This gives them the credibility they need to make them so compelling that they will spur readers on to action.

(e) It debunks some widely held beliefs that have been disproved by science.

Some of them are based on cherished folklore, others on dubious research sponsored by selfish business interests.

Where appropriate, I encourage readers to experiment—just as *I* did—to find solutions that fit their unique mix of needs and circumstances.

(f) It's presented in a time-saving form that makes it easy to grasp what's important. This is done with a direct, factual writing style liberally accentuated with typographical highlights.

c. When can you expect to reach your energy goal?

> *It's entirely possible that you will be able to get up immediately and with the greatest of ease already tomorrow morning.*

Ruth Tschudin, my wife, did it. She had, *for decades,* struggled for about an hour every day to get out of bed. But in the morning after having proofread the manuscript for my booklet <u>Wake Up to Abundant Energy: 113 Ways to Make it</u>

<u>Easy to "Rise and Shine"</u> she got up immediately, "just like that."

Merely reading that it is possible to get up at once was all it took Ruth to succeed (for reasons that will be explained later in this book).

> *Uncounted readers will be able to get up right away from now on, just as Ruth did.*

Others will succeed after minimal preparations, such as applying *only one* cherry-picked strategy such as:
• making an "attitude adjustment" (as per strategy No. 2), <u>or</u>
• foregoing the usual "nightcap" (No. 39), <u>or</u>
• banishing worrisome thoughts from their minds upon going to bed (No. 52).

Efforts like these may require only minutes of your time, but will enable you to sleep better and, consequently, wake up with surprisingly high energy.

But what will work best for you? There's no *one* superior way to proceed. What's ideal *for you* depends on aspects like the severity of your "energy problem," your health, habits, interests, ambitions, and—yes!—your motivation.

What and how much you should do depends also on *how much energy you want to gain*. So please don't try to accomplish too much too soon.

> *It's far better to make full use of most (if not all) of the strategies described in*

*this book because you'll benefit from
their combined energizing effects.*

d. How you will get the most out of this book

For most readers, the *best way* to proceed is as follows:

(a) READ the entire book, with pen in hand.

(b) COMPARE the recommended strategies with your
present lifestyle practices.

(c) "PERSONALIZE" the book. Underline, or add comments
in the margins. Highlight the information and
recommendations that are especially important to
you.

(d) START implementing all (or the highlighted) strategies.

(e) OBSERVE what happens as you go along. Notice the
way you feel.

(f) CELEBRATE your energy and mood gains.

(g) KEEP TRACK of your improvements by journaling, or
with check marks in the margins.

Take your present early-morning energy and mood levels into
consideration. *Don't be too much in a hurry* in your quest of
more energy and better mood. It's better to advance at a
sustainable pace than too quickly and failing.

Have confidence in your progress.
I'll show you exactly how to proceed.
I'll motivate and encourage you.
I'll prod you and will push you on.

If you occasionally get off course, go back to your agenda.

Persist until your new practices
have solidified into lifelong habits.

Enjoy the progress you'll be making on the way to greater vitality.

The changes will do wonders for how you feel and what you'll be able to accomplish.

Moreover, the journey will get steadily easier and better.

It will set a self-reinforcing
upward spiral in motion, with
success feeding on success.

No longer will you have to "start on empty" every day. Your weariness will wane. Your stamina will soar. Your mood and health will improve.

Your relationships, satisfaction and success on and off the job will reach new heights. You'll be delighted with your steady all-around progress and will enjoy experiencing how your life is taking on new meaning.

You'll be glad you took action
every time your alarm clock
breaks the stillness of the night.

So let's get going! Join me in the quest for greater vitality and superior quality of life.

> *Every major accomplishment —*
> *including energizing ourselves —*
> *begins in our brains.*

So we will start by conditioning our minds in certain very brain-specific ways.

Let's immerse ourselves right away into the all-important strategy No. 1.

PART II

YOUR P.E.P. (PERSONAL-ENERGY-POWER) ACTION PLAN

A. What to do now to start improving your energy, health, looks, success and satisfaction

1. Decide to wake up with lots of energy from this day forward

Major accomplishments are known to start in the space between our ears—in our brains. With clear decisions.

Empowering yourself to get out of bed promptly, easily and cheerfully, and with lots of energy to face the challenges and opportunities of the day ahead, is no exception.

Do you want to reach this goal? Are you willing to start thinking in certain new ways?

> *Are you ready to end your*
> *psychological fixation on fatigue?*

You probably are.

Or else you wouldn't read this book. So please just affirm to yourself right now:

> *"I've made up my mind. I'll wake*
> *up refreshed every morning from*
> *now on."*

Talking to yourself in this fashion—silently or out loud—may appear to be odd.

But do it anyway, for reasons that are well documented and will be fully explained later in this book.

For added impact, also *confirm in writing* that you've set yourself this goal.

You've made this *decision*. You *want* to wake up with all the energy you need all day long right from the beginning.

Also, enter this resolution in your agenda or diary, and on notes you'll display on your bathroom mirror and your computer monitor.

Believing this affirmation will get you to your energy goal sooner.

> *But there's no need for you to*
> *TRY to believe it.*

This is not "esoteric stuff" but based on both old *and* new psychological insights, as will also be explained later.

Your decision will manifest itself in due course as you are guided by the following proven procedures.

2. Banish negative self-talk from your life

I will never forget a motivational plaque I saw years ago. Placed on the oversized desk of an eminently successful executive, it read "JUST BEGIN! THE REST IS EASY."

Fortunately, our job here is a lot less difficult than the one of an executive facing a momentous, ever-changing mix of options.

Your goal is to gain so much energy that you have plenty of it even when you need it most: when it's time to get up.

So take the easy step No. 2. It marks the beginning of an *attitude adjustment leading to a new mindset.*

All it entails is to *stop—right this minute—making negative statements* about how you feel. Free yourself from the bonds of can't-do self-talk.

> *Stop saying to yourself:*
> - *"I wake up tired every morning."*
> - *"I'm always tired."*
> - *"I've been tired for years, and there's nothing I can do about it."*
> - *"It can only get worse."*

Such often-heard lamentations are *negative autosuggestions.*

When they trickle down to our powerful subconscious minds, they create *self-fulfilling prophecies of helplessness, gloom and failure.*

Again: we will have more to say later about how positive and negative autosuggestions work. For the time being, let's just note that making such "BAD" statements is a BAD habit that promotes BAD *psychological fixations on fatigue.*

The longer and more often we make them—silently or audibly— the more powerful they become, the more they sap our energy and depress our mood, and the harder it becomes for us to remove their negative effects from our lives.

3. Stop telling others how tired you are

Broadcasting our "energy problems" to those around us—perhaps hoping to elicit sympathy, or to impress them with our suffering— *is even worse:*

• It's a *negative autosuggestion* as well. We say it *and* hear it.

• It causes our listeners to respond in similarly negative terms, and gives birth to doom-reinforcing *"mutual-discouragement societies"*—groups of persons wallowing in energy-sapping gloom, self-pity, complaints and criticism whenever they get together.

• Our "negativity" may turn more positive-minded bystanders off and *mark us as toxic "complainers"* to stay away from.

In the world of business, we risk becoming known as individuals who are unfit for leadership, sales and other demanding positions ... because of our low energy, our pessimism and our demotivating effects on others.

4. Stop mindlessly answering "fine, thanks!"

Every time someone asks you "How are you?" you have an opening to shore up your prestige.

You're also getting a chance to lift not only *your* energy up to a higher level but also the energy of the person doing the asking.

Unless you're a hermit living in a barrel or on a mountain top you'll hear this question many times every day: at work ... at home ... at social gatherings ... in sports and on and on.

> *Don't let these golden opportunities*
> *slip away without making the most of*
> *them. Use them to make yourself and*
> *your counterparts feel happier and*
> *more alive.*

FIRST CONTEMPLATE the three major categories of responses.

Then consider using the one that serves you best.

When you become aware of their pros and cons, you may realize that your usual answer is not the best it could be, and that it should be replaced with a smarter choice.

We begin our review with the worst type of responses, then proceed to the ones that are so-so, and finally turn our attention to the very best—the ones that will be most beneficial to yourself and the persons you're with.

(1) COUNTERPRODUCTIVE ANSWERS

> *Rather pitiful are replies describing*
> *medical, family, financial or other*
> *problems you may have.*

Unless it's obvious that a "real" answer is expected (in which cases the question is usually more specific), the persons we encounter rarely want to be exposed to the depressing, energy-sapping litanies of other peoples' woes and their "negativity."

Moreover, whiners and complainers are considered to be socially inept. They are revealing their inability to cope with life's challenges, thus damaging their reputation and standing among those whose lives they touch.

Finally, they reinforce their own negative attitudes about themselves every time. But above all, they annoy the persons who ask them how they feel *just to be friendly*.

(2) TYPICAL, MEDIOCRE ANSWERS

"How are you?" is rarely an inquiry into our state of body and mind.

Not much better than the above are *the most commonly heard, lukewarm answers*—the ones that are neither clearly negative nor all that positive.

> *They are essentially meaningless,*
> *such as:*
> • *"Not bad."*

- *"Can't complain."*
- *"Hanging in there."*
- *"Okay, I guess."*

Such answers are somewhat improved by adding perfunctory counter-questions such as: "Thank you, *and you?"*

(3) STANDOUT ANSWERS

The most empowering response to "How are you?" is to *first put a friendly smile* on one's face (even if this takes a little effort when we're temporarily not our usual cheerful selves).

> *Then offer a cheerful comment such as:*
> - *"Wonderful!" (or "Great!" " Terrific!" "Fantastic!") Or:*
> - *"Couldn't be better!"Or:*
> - *"I'm doing great, and things are getting better all the time."*

Again, we may tag on something like *"Thanks for asking! And how are you?"* With such an addition, a superb complete answer might be:

> *"Thank you, John! It's going great and getting even better! And how's it going for you?"*

DO WE *HAVE* TO FEEL TERRIFIC IF WE *SAY* SO?

"Technically," we do, but for practical purposes it doesn't matter.

"How are you?" is rarely an inquiry into our state of body and mind. It's a formality—a mere "social lubricant."

Having enough problems of our own, most of us don't want to be burdened with other peoples' woes. But we decidedly want to be generous with warm, welcoming greetings.

HOW CAN WE GET THE MAXIMUM BENEFIT FROM OUR RESPONSES?

Spirited answers like "Just wonderful, thank you!" are far from meaningless. They create multiple heartening effects.

(1) *They energize us.* Validating the "fake-it-until-you-make-it" principle, they are quick-and-easy energy and mood "fixes."

As such, they are the do-it-yourself varieties of hypnotic suggestions. We know from medical and stage hypnotists that hypnotic suggestions tend to manifest themselves regardless of whether we believe them or don't.

(2) *They energize others.* They are infectious. At the very least, they make it far more pleasant for others to deal with us than with sad-sack self-proclaimed "victims of circumstances" who habitually dump their mental garbage on others.

Our positive self-declarations can even turn the mood and energy of entire groups of tired and grouchy persons around.

(3) *They bolster our prestige.* As manifestations of an upbeat, can-do spirit, they are among the hallmarks of success. They signal that we know how to deal with life's problems.

Projecting competence, they portray us as respected authorities.

(4) *They create a mystique.* Best of all, the people we encounter will wonder what magic powers we possess—what "secrets" enable us to triumph over problems and maintain a dynamic and effervescent spirit.

TRY THIS EXPERIMENT!

Especially if you believe that I've been exaggerating the benefits of the above "standout" answers, I challenge you to *dare* give one of them (such as "Great—couldn't be better, thank you, John, *and how do you feel today?*") a fair, non-prejudicial try.

> *Defy any inhibitions you may have to*
> *start projecting a more positive and*
> *more outgoing image from now on.*

Put your heart and soul into your responses, as follows.

Muster the *friendliest, most enthusiastic smile and tone of voice* you can conjure up (without going overboard, of course).

Your counterparts will at first be shocked, then wonder "what got into you." Then they will reward you with a smile of their own in return, and see you in a new light. You'll have gained in stature.

> *Unenthusiastic or inhibited*
> *individuals (and everybody else*
> *for that matter!) should practice*
> *being more outgoing and upbeat.*

They should habitually project more energy and happiness in every situation (not just when they're asked how they feel!) until their more genial, optimistic and self-assured demeanor has solidified into an empowering, enduring and endearing new habit.

Once this becomes "second nature," it's likely to increase their energy and enhance the atmosphere at their places of work and wherever else they meet other people.

> *Their transformation will mark a*
> *turning point in their own and*
> *other peoples' lives.*

It will dramatically improve how they feel about themselves, how they will be judged, and how successful they will be on the job and in their private lives.

....

An instructive footnote about smiling

A recent study *again* confirms the importance of presenting a friendly face to the world.

As reported in *Psychological Science*, researchers at Tufts University (Medford and Sumerville, Massachusetts) compared the facial expressions of the CEO's of the most profitable "Fortune-500" companies with the ones at the bottom of the list.

Their perceived likability turned out to be highly correlated with how people perceived their faces and the standing of their companies.

Thus, *smiling and "positivity"* apparently not only give those around us a "lift." They may even have the same effect on our employers' (and our own) earnings!

....

5. Snap out of gloom and doom—literally!

To enjoy success and high quality of life, we must perennially guard against "negativity." We shouldn't indulge in thoughts of being *doomed* to suffer from fatigue.

We should "cancel" mental rubbish right away so as not to get caught in downward spirals, and should *replace negative thinking with positive visions.*

A corny but practice-proven "trick" to accomplish this is to:
(a) wear a rubber band around *one* wrist, and
(b) use the *other* hand to let the band snap onto that wrist with enough force to cause some pain whenever we "catch" ourselves entertaining or spreading negative thoughts, and
(c) simultaneously command ourselves to *"snap out of it"*.

For best effect, we can follow up with a renewed commitment to uplifting thinking, such as:

> *"I will not fall into this trap again. I'm becoming more and more energetic, and have all the energy I need.*

Some readers may laugh at this procedure. That's quite all right with me. The "main thing" is that it is effective!

While making this simple "attitude modification," we may as well reinforce it by putting a *smile* on our faces.

6. Replace negative thinking with positive affirmations

Just trying to keep negative thoughts and beliefs out of one's mind rarely works. Nature "abhors a vacuum."

Counterproductive thinking will come back to haunt us unless we nip it in the bud to keep it away.

> *We need to replace mental rubbish*
> *immediately—as soon as it pops*
> *into our minds—with uplifting*
> *affirmations.*

But what's the best way to accomplish this?

We can use the time-honored formula coined by the famous French pharmacist-turned-psychologist-and-healer Emile Coué (1857-1926).

His all-purpose "mantra" has been used by hundreds of millions of people around the globe.

It has been employed with *often astonishing success* to improve health, energy, mood, habits and relationships.

Here it is. It's well worth memorizing and using daily:

> *"Day by day, in every way,*
> *I'm getting better and better."*

> *("Tous les jours, à tous points de*
> *vue, je vais de mieux en mieux.")*

In analogy to this world-famous autosuggestion, but focusing more narrowly on "fatigue fixations," we could, for instance, modify it to:

> *"I'm getting more and more energetic*
> *every morning when I wake up."*

7. Don't worry if you don't believe your autosuggestions

Autosuggestions are used to *create situations or conditions that do not exist when they are made.* Thus, you don't have to *believe* your affirmations to make them effective.

But if you believe them, they are likely to become effective sooner; in fact you've already put them into effect.

Repeating them will, however, strengthen them and make them more enduring.

> *The more you repeat affirmations,*
> *the more deeply they will sink into*
> *your subconscious mind, the more*
> *strongly they will attach themselves*

to it, and the sooner they will
manifest themselves in your life.

Presented in question-and-answer form, the following *background information* will lead to a fuller appreciation of the power of positive affirmations not only in raising our energy levels but also in improving virtually every other major aspect of our lives (such as health, weight control, relationships, happiness, and success in business and other endeavors).

The power of positive affirmations (self hypnosis) is so awesome, and the range of their application so wide, that they have evolved into *today's arguably most powerful "self-help success tools."*

....

Q+A: The subconscious mind's role in the success of high achievers

Please study this section even though it's more "technical" than other parts of this book. Gaining a basic understanding of the subconscious mind, hypnotism and related subjects is essential for attaining a sufficient appreciation of the often misunderstood and underused but awesome power of affirmations.

(a) How does self-hypnosis work?

Scientists still don't fully understand it. But—as pioneered by Emile Coué—self-hypnosis (which term is virtually the same as *autosuggestion*) can be used to turn the subconscious part of the mind into a self-improvement resource of awesome consequence.

(b) Who was Emile Coué?

Emile Coué (1857-1926) was a French pharmacist who evolved into a world-renowned psychologist and healer.

He had studied hypnosis at the University of Nancy, France.

After having observed that he could greatly improve the healing power of his medicines by extolling their beneficial effects to customers of his pharmacy, he became more and more fascinated by hypnosis.

Soon, he treated patients from all over the world to hypnosis free of charge.

When he could no longer keep up with demand, he developed *self-hypnosis* into a self-help method to improve health, vigor, mood, attitudes, habits, relationships, etc., and to get rid of all sorts of problems including insomnia, phobias, depression, pain, uncontrollable tremors, paralysis, bed-wetting, kleptomania, etc.

With self-hypnosis (autosuggestions), individuals were able to generate the same astonishing results as he and professional hypnotists could.

(c) What's the difference between affirmations and self-hypnosis, and what do they have in common with the subconscious mind?

Affirmations and self-hypnosis overlap:

• Affirmations are the "tools" used to achieve self-hypnosis.

• Self-hypnosis influences and shapes the subconscious mind (the part of our mental activities of which we are not consciously aware).

(d) Are *there any other manifestations that prove the power of the subconscious mind?*

Familiar to most of us are the feats performed by stage hypnotists.

But far more impressive is major surgery performed by Chinese country doctors using hypnosis and acupuncture for surgery rather than anesthesia.

Equally noteworthy as manifestations of the subconscious mind are phenomena as diverse as dreams, placebo healing effects, hallucinations, somnambulism (sleep walking), actions taken unknowingly in drunken stupor, as well as terror-induced paralyses, obsessive-compulsive acts, vertigo and mass hysteria.

(e) *Can we achieve the same results with willpower as with self-hypnosis?*

Once the subconscious mind has assimilated the ideas that were presented to it with repeated affirmations, it causes them to come to pass sooner or later.

For this to happen, *the will to make it happen must not be brought into play*. When the will and the subconscious mind collide, the subconscious mind invariably wins out.

Here is an example. If the subconscious mind tells us that we can't walk on a high wire, we won't be able to do so regardless of how much we want to do it.

We must first re-educate our subconscious minds with positive affirmations, and practice at increasing heights until "deep down" (in our subconscious minds) we "know" that we *can* do it.

(f) Which other approaches can have outcomes that are similar to the ones of negative or positive affirmations (autosuggestions)?

Of note among the NEGATIVE ones are curses, spells, witchcraft, shamanism, voodooism, mass hysteria and superstitions.

On the POSITIVE side are placebo effects, prayers (for healing and other needs), blessings, sacraments, ablutions, holy water, crosses and other religious symbols (including relics, pictures and statues of deities and saints, shrines), pilgrimages, self-exhorting pep talks, etc.

(g) Where are the limits of autosuggestions?

Success with self-hypnotic autosuggestions is limited only by the laws of nature. It is, for instance, impossible to heal broken bones within minutes, or to grow back amputated limbs.

But this still leaves huge untapped possibilities we can take advantage of in our daily lives.

(h) What are some recent popular sources of information on how we can benefit from positive affirmations?

We don't have to go back to Coué's writings for inspiration. His ideas and methods spawned, and have become part of, the contemporary self-help and self-improvement movement.

Authors like Norman Vincent Peale, Robert H. Schuller, and Joel Osteen have shown that we can accomplish far more than we ever dreamed of if we nurture our minds *and* take positive action. Noteworthy books include:

- *The Power of Positive Thinking* (Norman Vincent Peale, 1952),
- *Move Ahead with Possibility Thinking* (Robert H. Schuller, 1967), and
- *Your Best Life Now: 7 Steps to Living at Your Full Potential* (Joel Osteen, 2004).

....

8. Use affirmations at the right time

As already mentioned, positive affirmations should be used to squash negative thinking and feelings as soon as they come up.

In addition to using them defensively, we may want to slip them into our busy schedules as often as practical *throughout the day* to *keep ourselves moving forward on the right track.*

> *Coué recommended that we use positive affirmations at least twice a day:*
> - *upon waking up, and*
> - *from the time we go to bed until we lose ourselves in slumber.*

Ending the day with positive declarations is especially good advice because this is when we are between wakefulness and somnolence, thus in the state of mind that most closely resembles the one brought about by hypnosis, deep meditation or fervent prayer.

In other words, this is when our affirmations have particularly easy access to our subconscious minds.

To create an environment that is conducive to self-hypnosis *at any time* during the day, it's best to proceed as follows:
• Sit in a comfortable chair.
• Close your eyes.
• Relax the muscles throughout your body.
• Take a few slow, deep belly breaths.
• Then repeat your statements calmly and slowly as often as you wish, but at least three times.

9. Tailor affirmations to your personal needs

Some of us prefer shorter affirmations because they are easier to lull ourselves to sleep. Others may want to make them more specific—or more general. Or they may merely want them to sound more like themselves.

> *Examples:*
> • *"I sleep deeply, all night long."*
> • *"I wake up full of energy."*
> • *"Getting up is easy for me."*

Again, there's no need to limit yourself to affirmations relating to sleep, waking up, getting out of bed, and the like.

Make liberal use of other affirmations you create in line with *whatever need you have or goal you wish to reach.*

Formulate them positively and in the present tense:
• NOT "I *won't* be *nervous* any longer." BUT "I'm becoming (or "I *am*") calm and relaxed."
• NOT "My headache is disappearing" or "... fading away." BUT "My head is feeling better and better."

> *Here are some other examples:*
> • *"I'm taking it easy. I'm all right."*
> • *"I'm energetic and of good cheer."*
> • *"I have all the know-how I need, and I can do it."*
> • *"I'm getting more and more organized."*
> • *"When I'm up front to speak, I'm calm, poised and alert."*

10. Don't be concerned about the time required—you'll actually save time!

It took several pages to explain how we can *condition ourselves* to become "easy-risers."

This may have created the false impression that this transformation is very time-consuming.

Time is a rare commodity. We hardly ever appear to have enough of it. But we needn't be concerned here.

> *Fulfilling the previous recommendations*
> *will rarely take more than a few minutes.*

After all, they boil down to essentially this straightforward *modus operandi*:

- You stop bemoaning to yourself or others that you are fatigued and have difficulties "getting going" in the morning.

- You fight "negativity" of any type immediately with Coué's famous all-purpose affirmation (that bears repeating here):

  "Day by day, in every way,
  I'm getting better and better better."

Alternatively, create and use a "mantra" that is more to your liking.

While the entire process takes just a few minutes, it will save you the time you would otherwise lose in your struggle to get out of bed.

Without the right mindset and know-how, most people waste from 10 to 30 minutes (or more) until they manage to get up.

With the above procedures, you put this wasted time to far better use. Even more importantly, you can make getting up a pleasant experience rather than one you dislike or even hate and dread.

B. Techniques that will get you out of bed easily in five minutes or less

11. Forever banish the "Hardship-Wake-Up Scenario" from your life

CONGRATULATIONS! You've already come a long way. Up to now you have mainly accomplished the following:

- You *decided* to put an end to early-morning fatigue and misery.
- You *ended* your fixation on fatigue with autosuggestions easing your transition from sleep to wakefulness.

With this preparation, you're conditioned, and prepared, to take the logical next step *already tomorrow morning:*

> *When you wake up, get up using the surprisingly easy "Just-Do-It Approach."*

I'll explain the exact best procedure later.

It will enable you to get up promptly. Rising will cease to be a hassle even if your "early-morning experience" has—for decades—resembled the following ...

Sluggards' Sorry Scenario:

(a) Your alarm clock startles and annoys you. It "gets on our nerves," which is a stressful way of ushering in your day.

(b) You grope for the "darned thing" in the dark and possibly knock it over. You shut it off as soon as you find it.

(c) *You know you must get up now.* But feeling tired and somewhat depressed, you start negotiating with yourself.

Your internal dialog resembles the one that follows:

* *(Your alarm rings.)* "Ugh! Here we go! Time to get up! ... But I can stay a little longer, can't I?" *(You hit the "snooze" button.)*
* *(The alarm rings for the second time.)* "OK, I'd better move now. I don't want to get stuck in traffic! ... On the other hand, it's still a bit early." *(You hit the snooze button again.)*
* *(The alarm rings for the third time.)* "OK! OK! OK! ... I almost forgot: I still have to prepare for the nine-o'clock staff meeting ... I *really* have to get up now! ... Oh well! Maybe I'll feel better in ten more minutes." *(You "snooze" the alarm again.)*
* *(The alarm rings for the fourth time.)* "Whoa! I'm *REALLY* late now! ... But I'll just skip breakfast and will have a snack at the office instead."

In addition to being an inauspicious way of beginning the day, this scenario also extracts another heavy penalty.

We'll get back to this other highly undesirable consequence later.

But to gain a better understanding of the magnitude of the price we pay for lingering in bed, we first need to become more familiar with the mysterious state of mind and body called "sleep."

12. Use your knowledge of sleep to your advantage

Sleep has been defined as *a periodic state of rest for mind and body* that is usually characterized by: closed eyes, completely or partially lost consciousness, decreased bodily movement, reduced responsiveness to external stimuli, and a certain type of brain-wave activity.

> *Although sleepers are supposed to be resting, they undergo a surprising number of complex processes.*

One of them is a pattern of *brain-wave cycles and stages.*

With a basic knowledge of these phenomena we can make more enlightened decisions regarding sleep and its effects on the energy we have upon waking up in the morning.

Every night, the average sleeper passes through ABOUT 5 SLEEP CYCLES of around 70 to 90 minutes each, and each sleep cycle consists of 5 SLEEP STAGES:

- STAGE 1 (4 to 5% of every cycle) is characterized by drowsiness and drifting in and out of sleep.

- STAGE 2 (45 to 55%) is light sleep during which brain waves, breathing and heart rate are slowing down.

- STAGE 3 (4 to 6%) marks the onset of delta brain waves and deep sleep.

- *STAGE 4 (12 to 15%) is the deepest, most therapeutic cycle*, with delta-wave activity. Delta brain waves are very slow and usually associated with the *unconscious mind*.

• STAGE 5 (20 to 25%) is Rapid-Eye Movement (REM) Sleep, marked by jerking of eyes, occurrence of *dreams* and acceleration of brain waves to the wakefulness level.

If we don't get enough *Deep (Stage-4) Sleep* because of a full stomach or for any other reason (such as noise, insufficiently dark bedroom, jet lag, sleep apnea, restless-leg syndrome, snoring by a bedmate, etc.), we will invariably wake up tired in the morning, and are likely to remain tired all day long.

> *As the night progresses, the periods of shallower Stage-5-REM Sleep get longer and longer while the periods of the more invigorating No.4-Deep Sleep become shorter and shorter.*

Thus, *"sleeping in"* can be a big (perhaps pleasant) waste of time. It's just not very invigorating!

> *In addition, resting in bed longer over the weekend interrupts our sleep pattern and is the most important cause of the Monday-morning hangovers.*

Even though REM Sleep is far less important than Deep Sleep, REM Sleep is by no means immaterial.

According to very recent research, sleepers who are deprived of REM sleep don't get the *full* benefit of a good night's sleep.

Now that these technicalities are settled—at least for us here but certainly not for sleep researchers—let's go back to the Hardship Wake-Up Scenario and its shockingly high price tag.

13. Stop paying the high price of tarrying in bed

The Hardship (Procrastination) Wake-Up Scenario described above is far more detrimental than most of us realize.

ONE, it prolongs the agony. Remaining in bed and trying—but failing—to get up reasonably soon is depressing, and often sets a *foul mood* for the entire day.

TWO, it creates or reinforces a negative self-image. We may perceive ourselves as weaklings and failures. This is demoralizing.

THREE, the extra time spent under cover fails to generate an "energy bonus." It can't rev us up because the Deep-Sleep phases of the nightly sleep cycles (around five for most individuals, as mentioned above) are getting more and more shallow as the night progresses.

> *We simply can't get into the most productive periods of energizing Deep Sleep when morning approaches. We will, at best, drift in and out of episodes of shallow slumber.*

FOUR, remaining in bed squanders our most precious resource: time.

Facilitated by the repeated use of the insidious "snooze" features of most alarm clocks, "just ten more minutes" expands easily into 30, 60 or even more minutes of wasted time every morning.

> *Sadly, we permit the time-wasting*
> *habit of lingering in bed to continue*
> *for years even though we keep*
> *lamenting about "never having*
> *enough time!"*

14. Gain one full month's worth of work time every year

The waste of time (the "stuff that life is made of" according to Benjamin Franklin) caused by the above scenario is stunning.

Let's do the math!

In 365 days of dilly-dallying in bed for an average of *30 minutes*, we lose 365 half-hours, thus 182.5 hours. This is slightly more than 4.5 forty-hour work weeks (because 4.5 times 40 hours totals 180 hours).

> *Thus, giving up procrastinating in*
> *bed for 30 minutes every morning is*
> *tantamount to gaining more than one*
> *"bonus work month" every year!*

And no longer wasting an *entire hour* equals more than *two* extra months a year.

> *For many of us, rising without delay is*
> *the best way to tap our single largest*

> *"time reserve"* — *the squandered intervals*
> *between waking up and getting out of bed.*

But can we *really* get ourselves to rise promptly when the alarm clock rings?

YES, WE CAN!

Chances are excellent *even if* we:
• have suffered from severe early-morning distress for a long time,
• have repeatedly tried, and failed, to come to grips with this problem,
• believe to be stuck with it for life, and
• are convinced that it can only get worse as we get older.

The fact is we're not stuck. We can get up right away as early as tomorrow morning as we'll see next.

15. Use the stunningly easy "Just-Do-It Approach"

As the term denotes, this approach boils down to just making it happen.

This may appear to be ludicrous to individuals for whom getting up has been a troublesome, tough struggle for as long as they can remember. But it can be done *even at first try.*

The "Just-Do-It Approach" gets its astonishing power from the age-old *"Action Principle"*:

"JUST DO IT, AND YOU'LL HAVE THE POWER."

Here's an example. Giving up nicotine is believed to be extremely difficult.

But my father-in-law did it "just like that." He gave up a 40-cigarettes-a-day addiction from one moment to the next. He spontaneously threw the remaining "cigs" into the garbage and never smoked another cigarette again for the rest of his life.

When friends and colleagues asked him how he accomplished this feat, he said "I just did it. It was no big deal."

Likewise, British book author *Allen Carr*—who was afraid of dying from lung cancer—kicked a 100-cigarettes-a-day habit after 31 years, also from one moment to the next. He was motivated by fear of imminent death. To his great surprise, he didn't have any problems as a result, either.

Mr. Carr described this accomplishment in *The Allen Carr Easy Way to Quit Smoking.*

This rather thin book was first published in 1985, and has been bought by tens of millions of smokers around the world.

In the book, he made just three major points:

(a) "I quit without nicotine gum, patches, inhalers, injections or hypnosis."

(b) "I had no problems as a result:
• no suffering from withdrawal symptoms,
• no difficulties coping with stress,
• no loss of pleasure."

(c) "Therefore, dear reader, do as I did: JUST QUIT!"

This was Carr's entire "system." It had an astonishing 90-percent success rate (based on a three-month money-back guarantee for participants in his half-day seminars).

Ruth Tschudin (my wife) formerly languished in bed for about one extra hour every day until she finally managed to emerge from her bed. But she got up *at once* in the morning after having proofread the manuscript of my booklet <u>Wake Up to Abundant Energy: 113 Ways to Make it Easy to "Rise and Shine"</u>.

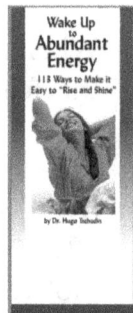

> *Overcoming bad habits, fear or*
> *anything we want to give up by*
> *"just doing it" is the preeminent*
> *life strategy of highly successful*
> *individuals.*

Try it tomorrow morning! Get up immediately when the alarm rings—without giving it another thought. JUST DO IT!

You'll be surprised by how easy it is to do what was formerly impossible for you: to rise promptly without getting into drawn-out arguments with yourself.

> *Congratulations are in order if you
> did just that. You validated the
> awesome power of "just doing it!"*

And having succeeded once, you know that you can do it again and again.

In the unlikely worst case—if this straightforward approach doesn't work for you as expected—you can pat yourself on the back for having tried. And you can try the same approach again later, or—better— use one of the following *more gradual* strategies.

16. Alternatively, use the two-minute "No-Sweat Method"

You may be curious about *my* early-morning ritual. *I could easily get on my feet immediately* upon waking up at 5:25 a.m. (summoned, by the way, only by my *"mental* alarm clock"). But I don't get up that quickly.

> *I spend two additional minutes in
> bed to ease into my daytime action
> mode ... by using my three-step
> "No-Sweat Method."*

To use this easy-as-1-2-3 way of greeting the new day, proceed as follows *already tomorrow morning*.

The description is detailed to make it easy to understand, appreciate and apply. But the entire procedure—from the time you wake up to the time when you're "up and at it"—*will take only two minutes*.

(a) TAKE FIVE SLOW, DEEP "BELLY BREATHS."

In less than half a minute, "belly-breathing" will re-energize your body and mind by eliminating carbon dioxide and other fatigue-inducing waste products from your cells and bringing their oxygen supply to daytime-action-ready levels.

You'll be amazed at how much this procedure will invigorate you if you follow these proven guidelines:

• BREATHE "WITH YOUR BELLY"—the lower part of your lungs, where most of your blood circulates. (Don't breathe with your chest and shoulders. "Puffed-chest breathing" is inefficient.)

• CHECK YOURSELF. To see if you're doing it right, place one hand just below the rib cage. You are breathing efficiently if your hand is pushed forward, and if it feels as if your belly is filling with air like a balloon when you inhale, and the hand goes back in when you exhale.

• INHALE slowly through your nose, while silently (or audibly) declaring "in with energy!"

• EXHALE even more slowly through your mouth, saying "out with fatigue!"

• DON'T OVERDO IT. Don't risk getting dizzy. Breathe slowly, deeply and in a relaxed way.

• DO IT NOW: To apply this technique properly tomorrow morning, *practice it at once*, and then again later today. You'll love its stimulating effect.

> TIP: *Use deep-breathing also*
> *repeatedly throughout the day to*
> *fight daytime fatigue.*

(b) STRETCH YOURSELF.

Gently stretch your muscles. Extend yourself "in all directions" for about a minute to give your energy another boost:

• Stretch your arms and legs and then relax them. Similarly, spread and then bend your fingers and toes upward and then down a few times. Afterwards, relax these digits as well.

• Pull your shoulders back, and push the "hollow" middle part of your back forward so that your belly sticks out.

Flexing and relaxing increases the circulation of your blood (with energizing oxygen in it) throughout your body, and will feel "just wonderful."

But beware: Start every stretching movement gently, so as not to hurt any muscles or tendons. Then intensify it gradually without overdoing it.

(c) EXPRESS YOUR GRATITUDE.

Silently (or audibly) express your gratitude for: your ability to walk, see, hear, etc. ... the roof above your head ... your education ... your (overabundant!) food ... the love and support of your family and friends ... the privilege of living in our great country, etc.

These "positives" in our lives usually more than offset the "negatives" (such as difficulties at work ... financial losses ... minor illnesses, etc.).

Focusing on the many good aspects of our lives prepares us *mentally* for a great day.

> *After this three-step preparation,*
> *you're ready to get up. Rise!*

17. For even greater ease, go for the "Five-Minute Method"

This is the early-morning strategy of choice for individuals wishing to move to wakefulness at an *extra-comfortable pace.*

Rather than getting up in two minutes, they spend three more minutes to go through my leisurely *seven-step action sequence.*

> *Because the steps are extremely*
> *low, climbing from one to the next*
> *is almost effortless.*

Even severely energy-challenged individuals can do it readily and easily.

After having silenced the alarm clock, please proceed as follows:

(a) Take five "belly breaths.

"Belly-breathing was already explained before. But we'll repeat the "essentials" here for your convenience.

Take five slow, deep breaths using mostly the bottom part of your lungs (rather than the far less efficient top) to breathe.
* *When you inhale,* the abdomen expands forward and downward while you affirm "energy in!" (which creates a somewhat self-hypnotic effect).
* *When you exhale,* it retracts, and you say "fatigue out!"

This procedure expels carbon dioxide and other waste products from your body and replaces them with *energizing oxygen.*

(b) Express your gratitude.

To put your *mind* on a positive track, take about one minute to remind yourself of some of your blessings. As mentioned earlier, they include your mobility, the possession of your five senses, your shelter, the support you're getting from those around you, the opportunities we have in our free society, etc.

> *By focusing on these "positives," you are*
> *taking an easy second step to prepare your-*
> *self MENTALLY for another great day.*

(c) Smile to yourself.

Smile *even though nobody will see it* in the darkness of your bedroom.

Because of the connectivity between your facial muscles and the hypothalamus (one of the brain's major pleasure centers), this third step will push your mind even more toward an *empowering* feeling of happiness.

(d) Wiggle your toes.

Exercise them as follows:
• Slowly bend them upward while belly-breathing in through your nose.
• Then slowly curl them down as you exhale through your mouth.

This is a minimal effort. (Laugh if you wish; laughing is good for you!) But this exercise is helpful for individuals who are still groggy at the beginning of this fourth stage. It *starts* the process of *setting their bodies in motion.*

(e) Stretch your muscles.

Spread your arms and legs, and hands and toes. Pull your shoulders back and stick out your chest. Extend yourself in all directions; stretch all major muscle groups. This will give your energy an additional boost.

Begin every movement gently.

Then gradually increase your muscle tension until you feel refreshed throughout your body. This is an indication that your *increased blood circulation* has flushed carbon dioxide and other fatigue-inducing waste material out of your body tissue and replaced them with revitalizing oxygen.

(f) RISE!

After *no more than five minutes* of preparation, you're now ready, and *you "JUST DO IT!"*

You can sit up and turn to the side of the bed. Or get up with a swiveling sideway motion. Then plant your feet an the floor, and start walking—slowly if necessary to avoid dizziness.

(g) Let there be light!

Open the curtain, or let electric light flood the room. The light will hit the photosensitive cells of the retina (which is located in the back of our eyes). This will *stop the secretion of melatonin* by the brain's pineal gland.

Now you're no longer under the influence of the "sleep hormone." *Congratulations!* With this seventh step, you've completed the transition to daytime readiness.

> *You made getting up a "snap"*
> *rather than the drawn-out*
> *anguish it used to be.*

To master the transition from night to day, you divided. To solve your problem, you broke it up into seven practically effortless baby steps.

> *Now, after having validated the*
> *procedure, getting out of bed in*
> *the morning will never again be*
> *the predicament it used to be.*

From now on, every day can be a positive experience *right from the start.*

C. What you can do in the afternoon to make getting up easy in the following morning

18. Stop consuming caffeinated products by mid-afternoon

To enjoy energy-restoring sleep, we need to consider that caffeine is a powerful *central-nervous-system excitant.*

We must stop consuming coffee and other stimulating products well before the day's end.

> *Cutting off caffeine around 3:00 p.m. appears to be a "no-brainer" for most, but not all, of us.*

In rare individuals, caffeine has a *totally sleep-defying effect for up to and over 10 hours.*

Astonishingly, some individuals can use caffeinated coffee as a *sleep aid (!).*

> *Because the effects of caffeine vary so much from individual to individual, coffee-drinkers may want to experiment to determine their personal best caffeine-quitting time."*

Caffeine is present not only in non-decaf coffee but to varying degrees also in *other beverages* including *tea* and many *soft drinks* as well as in some food products (see chart below).

The caffeine content differs also *within* product categories. In coffee, for instance, the caffeine depends on: (1) the type of coffee beans used, (2) how they're roasted and (3) how the beverage is prepared (e.g. brewed, drip, etc.).

Coffee statistics are not consistent. But here are representative data gleaned from the Center for Science in the Public Interest, The EnergyFiend Database, and CNN.

....

PRODUCT	CAFFEINE IN MILLIGRAMS
COFFEE	
Generic, brewed (8 oz.)	135 (range: 80-200)
Starbucks Grande (16 oz.)	320
Dunkin' Donuts, regular (16 oz.)	206
Instant, generic (8 oz.)	95 (range: 27-173)
Espresso, generic (2 oz.)	80 (range: 60-180)
TEA	
Black, brewed (1 tea bag)	55 (range: 40-100)
Snapple, Lemon (16 oz.)	42
Green tea (1 tea bag)	20 (range: 18-30)
SOFT DRINKS	
The FDA limits cola and pepper soft drinks to 71 mg per 12 oz.	
Pepsi (12 oz.)	38
Diet Pepsi (12 oz.)	36
Coca-Cola Classic (12 oz.)	35
7-Up, Regular or Diet (12 oz.)	0

ENERGY DRINKS
Spike Shooter (8.4 oz.)   300
Red Bull (8.3 oz.)   80

FROZEN DESSERTS
Ben & Jerry's Coffee Heath Bar   84
   Crunch (8 fl. oz.)

Haagen-Dazs Coffee Ice   58
   Cream (8 fl. oz.)

CHOCOLATE, CANDY
Jolt Caffeinated Gum (1 stick)   33
Hershey Chocolate Bar (1.55 oz.)   9

OVER-THE-COUNTER DRUGS
NoDoz Max. Strength (1 tablet)   200
Excedrin Extra Strength (2 tabs.)   130
Anacin Maximum Strength (2 tabs.)   64

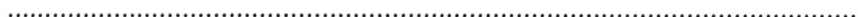

....

Is caffeine good for your health?

This question continues to be controversial. So pick the answer you like best, in line with your taste preferences and the following pros and cons.

Lately—especially since 2012—studies favoring coffee consumption have become more numerous. This may be due to intensified initiatives of the powerful global coffee lobby (which is a major sponsor of such studies).

Another possible explanation may be recent efforts of the food-supplement industry to launch green-coffee extracts to improve blood-sugar control.

While test results are far from uniform, many have come to the conclusion that *consuming 200 to 300 mg of caffeine per day* (which is what we get in somewhat more than two 8-oz. cups of generic coffee) *is harmless* and may even be beneficial because of coffee's antioxidant effects.

But drinking more than 500 mg (approximately four to five cups and up) often causes irritability, nervousness, anxiety, irregular heartbeat, diarrhea, vomiting, dizziness, headaches and *insomnia* (which is, in itself, one of the major causes of fatigue).

Like most other drugs, caffeine also causes *undesirable side effects*. It can increase cholesterol, raise blood pressure, damage blood vessels and cause heart and stomach problems.

Moreover, coffee should be avoided during pregnancy.

Further complicating the complex picture, frequently-used coffee additives such as sugar, many sugar substitutes, cream, creamer (as well as the saturated and trans fats, artificial colors, flavors and the preservatives that creamers sometimes contain) make many caffeinated "javas" decidedly injurious to our health.

As shown in the next chapter, this is not the end of the caffeine/coffee "story" because other widely consumed products contain caffeine as well.

19. Be prudent with medications containing caffeine

It's common knowledge that the consumption of coffee, tea, certain soft drinks, chocolate, etc., late in the day, is likely to sabotage our sleep.

But many of us don't realize that *medications* should be scrutinized for their caffeine content as well.

Of the hundreds of NON-PRESCRIPTION MEDICATIONS (also called over-the-counter, or OTC, medications) commonly found in drug, food, convenience, department and other stores, many contain at least 30 milligrams of caffeine.

Excedrin Extra Strength, for instance, delivers 130 mg per maximum-recommended two-tablet dose. Midol Menstrual Maximum Strength Caplets contain 60.

Among PRESCRIPTION MEDICATIONS, the ones based on ergotamine are "loaded" with caffeine. Migergot suppositories and Cafergot tablets contain 100 mg each.

Prescription *and* non-prescription ANALGESICS (pain relievers) are also frequently complemented with caffeine.

Why? For two good reasons. Caffeine activates the analgesics more quickly (bringing us faster relief), and makes them 40 percent more powerful (permitting a reduction of the analgesic content).

Noteworthy in addition to caffeinated analgesics are caffeinated *pharmaceuticals with fatigue-inducing* ANTIHISTAMINES as active ingredients (such as many medications providing relief from ALLERGIES, COLDS and FLU).

WARNING. The *combined use* of various types of caffeinated drinks, foods and drugs is dangerous because of their *cumulative effects.*

Especially perilous is the consumption of such drugs by patients ingesting more than about 500 mg of caffeine per day in coffee, tea, soft drinks, cocoa/chocolate and other food products and drinks.

Reminder: four or five cups of coffee alone contain about 500 mg of caffeine.

> *Therefore:*
> - *Scrutinize beverage, food and drug labels for caffeine.*
> - *Avoid caffeinated medications after mid-afternoon if this does not create any other health risks.*
> - *Ask your doctor or pharmacist for caffeine-free alternatives whenever this is practical.*

20. Quit smoking

Another stimulant—but far more insidious than caffeine—is nicotine, an alkaloid found mostly in *tobacco* and *coca* plants.

On the POSITIVE side, nicotine melts away anxiety, relaxes body and mind, and nevertheless enhances energy and alertness. An appealing, seemingly contradictory mix of benefits!

But the NEGATIVES of nicotine outweigh what's good about it by a huge margin. Nicotine is highly addictive.

The addiction creeps up on smokers and is widely believed to be one of the hardest to break (but see No. 15 above about a surprisingly effective strategy to quit smoking).

Nicotine is absorbed by *active and passive smoking* as well as by *chewing and sniffing* tobacco products. All of these forms of consumption make the heart race, elevate blood pressure, lead to circulatory disease and cancel the invigorating effects of sleep.

> *Nicotine addicts can hardly ever*
> *get enough sleep because of the*
> *onset of withdrawal symptoms.*

Here is how this develops. When the body's nicotine supply gets low—usually sometime after midnight—the brain pushes addicts to replenish it. The cravings drive them to either *get up* to smoke, or even to *smoke in bed*.

In either case, they will wake up in the morning with a *hangover*. Worse still, smokers often contract *lung, oral or throat cancer* sooner or later.

One of every two smokers dies as a consequence of smoking (often gasping for air much like persons who are drowning).

Particularly at risk are aficionados who also consume *alcohol*. The combination of caffeine and alcohol can be devastating.

21. Take exercise breaks

Persons experiencing mid-afternoon energy slumps (and that's most of us!) face a dilemma.

To keep going, they may "need" caffeine. But if they get it in one form or another, they may have difficulties falling asleep at bedtime. Or their sleep will be shallow and fitful, and they'll wake up tired in the following morning and are likely to suffer from low energy all day long.

Fortunately, there's a caffeine-free solution. We can take *exercise breaks* to increase our intake of energizing oxygen and improve the circulation of the oxygen-enriched blood in the body and brain.

> *Paradoxically, exercising is the most*
> *effective way of boosting our energy*
> *when we're tired (but not when*
> *we're totally exhausted).*

Exercise is also the best way to make it easy for us to fall asleep at bedtime, and to sleep well throughout the night.

Reason: Exercise makes us *physiologically* tired, not tired from stress (which makes Deep Sleep hard to come by).

Mid-afternoon may not be the right time for *vigorous workouts.* But you may be able to overcome the doldrums by:
* repeating positive affirmations (above, No. 6),
* doing some deep-breathing exercises (No. 16),
* short walks—if necessary just to the office water cooler, but preferably outdoors in broad daylight, or

• a combination of some of these approaches (such as deep-breathing and repeating positive affirmations while walking outdoors).

We can do much more to boost our energy than merely take exercise *breaks,* as shown in the following chapters.

D. How to leave your workday worries and daytime stress behind so as not to sabotage your sleep

22. Find "closure" for workday worries and frustrations

Work is a major source of security and satisfaction. It's also a breeding ground of worries and frustrations that can spill over into "our own time" in the evening and keep us awake at night.

> *To maintain our energy, we can't*
> *permit job-related troubles to spill*
> *into our private lives.*

Here's a good way to accomplish this before leaving one's place of work:
* Review your day's work and *take note of your positive accomplishments* of any kind, large and small. Do so while maintaining a sense of satisfaction.
* Don't worry about the tasks that are left undone. Instead, *put them on a To-Do-List for the following day.*
* *Leave the list,* and whatever concerns it may embody, at the place of work, to be tackled there on the following day.

Finally, enlist the power of the subconscious mind. Use an affirmation such as:

> *"Now I can take it easy. I'm relaxed*
> *and feeling better and better."*

23. Skip the so-called "happy hour"

What else can you do, after a stressful workday, to reduce tension and smooth the transition to the well-deserved leisure mode?

Should you join the "happy-hour" crowd in the convivial atmosphere of a cozy bar or pub? Or would you rather enjoy a soothing drink or two at home?

Regardless of the locale, alcohol-based "attitude adjustments" have advantages and drawbacks.

As a sedative, alcohol "calms the nerves." It can be a pleasing prelude to a delightful evening. And when it's time to go to bed, it can make falling asleep a piece of cake.

But, on balance, the *disadvantages* of alcohol consumption after work outweigh the benefits by a huge margin. They are similar to the ones of smoking.

> *Even moderate alcohol intake up to six hours prior to bedtime can have unfortunate consequences for the duration and quality of sleep during the second half of the night.*

This is when the alcohol's sedative effect is wearing off and yields to *pernicious aftereffects*.

Sleep becomes increasingly shallow. *We don't get enough, or any, Deep Sleep* (Stage-4 Sleep) during which mind and body perform most of their nightly repair work. Consequently:
• Sleep becomes more and more fitful.

- *We wake up sometime after midnight* (often repeatedly).
- *Even though we may be exhausted, returning to sleep will be challenging if not impossible.

Among the usual aftereffects are *hangovers*, extreme *difficulties getting up, daytime fatigue* and reduced alertness, danger of causing *accidents* on the road and at work, *irritability* and its attendant *social problems* (such as not getting along well with family members, colleagues, customers, etc.), as well as loss of employment, advancement, earnings and other opportunities.

Moreover, drinking a daily glass or shot (or two) usually starts out innocently enough.

But, more often than is commonly believed, it gradually leads to diminishing effects of alcohol on the body (resulting from the body's "down regulation"), and consequently ever in-creasinging *alcohol consumption and addiction.*

Tragically, most drinkers believe to be in control of themselves while they're on their way down that slippery slope.

24. Set the stage for a delightful evening

Rather than merely leaving work-related concerns behind, or drowning them in alcohol, we can *get ready to truly enjoy* the leisure time that lies ahead *by thinking ahead.*

> *On the way home, reflect on
> how you can make the evening a
> pleasant experience for yourself
> and those around you.*

How can you turn it into a *happy prelude to a night of energizing sleep?*

The possibilities are virtually unlimited. To illustrate, here are some random *questions* you could ask yourself:

• Can I bring something with me as a token of affection?

• Should I just display a friendly smile, or offer a tender hug or a heartfelt compliment?

• What *specific* compliment would be appropriate and much appreciated?

• Am I prepared to listen to the concerns of my "significant other" before I burden him or her with my own?

• Should I suggest that we go for a walk or engage in some other light exercise for a pleasant change of pace?

• Should we perhaps play a relaxing game?

• Can we discuss an *uplifting* subject (such as: how to help someone cope with a problem, what to do during an upcoming weekend, or where to spend the next vacation)?

• Is there anything else that's more meaningful than indiscriminately watching the "boob tube"?

• Or should I just enjoy some delightful "me-time," either listening to great music, curling up in my favorite easy chair with a great book, building a model airplane, or whatever?

E. Powerful energy-enhancing actions you can take right after work

25. Exercise your sleep and energy problems away

Validating the results of countless older studies, researchers at the Stanford University School of Medicine in California confirmed that *exercise is a superior way to facilitate falling asleep and getting more sleep,* especially more *Deep Sleep* (Phase-4 Sleep).

> *Exercise is the best-possible "sleep aid."*

In spite of its great value, exercise doesn't have to cost any money. You can do it at home, without any special equipment.

It addition to increasing our general state of health and improving how we feel and look it has *remarkably positive "side effects"* on how well we sleep.

Here is how the Stanford researchers came to this conclusion.

They had 54- to 75-year-old sedentary adults with mild sleep complaints exercise at least four times a week. On two days, they engaged them in aerobic group exercises for 30 minutes. And on two more days, they had them individually do 40 minutes of brisk walking or stationary-bicycle pedaling.

At the end of their 16-week program, the results were astonishing. On average, it took participants only 15 minutes to nod off (which was half as much time as before the research program began), and they were able to sleep 45 minutes longer.

26. Give exercise a higher "mindshare"

To stay motivated to give exercise its proper place in our busy lives, keep these two major causes of its the sleep-enhancing effects in your mind:

• *Exercise results in physiological fatigue.* The brain compensates for it by increasing the need for sleep—especially the most therapeutic *Deep Sleep.* (In contrast, *stress-induced* sleep makes it difficult if not impossible for us to get enough of this Stage-4 Sleep.)

• *Exercise raises body temperature.* This induces a subsequent drop to a lower nighttime body temperature. This drop, in turn, promotes sleep.

Regrettably, most of us don't exercise enough to: (1) cause our temperature to rise and then fall sufficiently, and (2) experience healthy (physiological) fatigue.

Thus, we are neither tired enough *physically,* nor do we benefit from a subsequent temperature drop that would promote sleep. Consequently, many of us don't get the sleep we need to wake up energized—*even if we spend excessive lengths of time in bed.*

> *85 percent of Americans believe they*
> *are getting enough exercise. But only*
> *25 percent actually do.*

For this reason and because of the many beneficial effects of physical activity on our sleep and our general health, taking a closer look at these effects is eminently worthwhile.

Regular and *sufficiently vigorous* exercise can help us to:
* *reduce stress* (by removing lactic acid from our blood),
* *boost energy*, stamina and endurance (by strengthening our heart and circulatory system),
* *improve mood* (by increasing the secretion of "feel-good hormones" like epinephrine and endorphins),
* sharpen memory, thinking, reasoning and alertness (by increasing the brain's oxygen supply),
* *keep us slim* and win the "battle of the bulge" (by using up calories if combined with proper nutrition),
* *slow down aging* (by preventing muscle loss, retaining joint mobility and bone density), and
* *enjoy more and better sex* (by stimulating blood production and circulation, increasing the secretion of sexual hormones and feel-good endorphins, and improving body self-image).

For reasons that are too numerous to mention here, exercise can also help us to:
* *strengthen the immune system* and keep a multitude of health threats at bay,
* *increase "good" high-density cholesterol* and decrease "bad" low-density cholesterol,
* *prevent and treat chronic illnesses* such as heart disease, high blood pressure, type-2 diabetes, obesity, stroke, breast, prostate and other cancers, Alzheimer's, insomnia, depression, etc., and
* *feel healthier and look better.*

> *Exercise is a necessity for sleeping*
> *well, increasing one's energy and*

*vitality, becoming and remaining
healthy, and slowing down aging.*

In eons of evolution, mankind was genetically programmed to make tremendous efforts to hunt down barely enough food for survival. But in our modern civilization, most of us have all-too-easy access to far-too-many calories with minimal physical effort.

This gap between our genetic inheritance and today's sedentary lifestyle has brought about an unprecedented epidemic of obesity and other chronic illnesses.

*Coupled with good nutrition,
exercise is the best way to escape
the downside of today's couch-
potato civilization.*

27. Exercise at least 30 minutes a day

To get a superior night's sleep and wake up with high energy, we need to exercise almost every day. But ...

*There's plenty of evidence that
30 to 60 minutes of moderately
intense exercise on at least four
days a week is adequate to
maintain good health.*

Exercising longer and with greater intensity will improve our performance. But it is unlikely to benefit our health substantially.

It also increases our exposure to *exercise risks* (such as injuries of muscles, joints and bones of runners; injuries of persons with serious cardiovascular and other chronic illnesses; etc.).

Individuals who "can't find 30 minutes a day"—one forty-eighth of our time—to keep their bodies in reasonably good condition, need to reassess their values, goals and preferences.

Do you just not have any time for exercise after work?

Then how about exercising beforehand? How about getting up half an hour earlier? (By the way, most individuals overestimate the length of the sleep they need.)

What's better: exercising early in the morning, or in the afternoon or evening?

Research studies disagree on this subject. No studies have proven conclusively which time of day is best. So here you're on your own.

Some of us prefer exercising—at home or at a health club—before going to work. They want to rev up their energy in the morning, or just "get the exercise out of the way." Others favor evenings. Again others prefer exercising around noontime.

> *There's no use agonizing over the objectively best time for training. Any time will be suitable. JUST DO IT!*

More important than your timing is only that you exercise *regularly*.

There are, however, two major exceptions:

* One is that strenuous exercise should, for many of us, *end about three hours prior to bedtime* to give the body enough time to calm down. We don't want to get our adrenaline flowing and our heart racing when we go to bed.

* The other exception is that we should never exercise *less than two hours after a full meal*. Going for a leisurely walk would, however, aid the digestive process and help us to unwind.

28. Consider the many great exercise options (Q and A)

Exercise at any suitable time of day is indispensable for individuals who want to begin their waking hours with an abundance of energy.

An overview of the vast subject of exercising would exceed the scope of this book. But it may be useful to remind ourselves of some of the most essential facts.

Here are some of the *questions to be considered* in setting up a suitable exercise program. The answers should make it easy to come up with a fitness routine that will match your personal needs and circumstances.

(a) Which are the two major types of exercise to choose from?

AEROBIC EXERCISES (such as walking, running, aerobic dancing, cross-country skiing, swimming, bicycling, stepping, tennis) strengthen the lungs and heart and make the heart pump blood faster.

These workouts also boost the number of red blood cells (which increases the circulation of life-enhancing oxygen). In addition, they pump the oxygen-laden blood more forcefully throughout the body (which raises our energy) and stimulate the production of endorphins (hormones that make us feel good).

STRENGTH EXERCISES (such as weight or resistance training) require our muscles to exert a force against the resistance provided by free weights, exercise machines or elastic bands.

> *Without strength training, we lose*
> *up to one-half pound of muscle*
> *mass every year beginning in our*
> *mid-twenties.*

In addition to *preserving* muscle mass, strength training helps us to *increase* it (within the limits put upon us by our genes) and to control body fat (if we also eat well). Thus, ...

> *Strength training serves to "sculpt"*
> *good-looking physiques.*

It also reduces our risk of injury by strengthening joints, tendons and the muscles surrounding them.

(b) Which types of exercise are best for us?

Any activity that deserves to be called physical exercise not only contributes to our health and well-being, but also increases the energy with which we begin, and continue, our waking hours.

But a *combination* of aerobic exercises and strength training is the best way to:

* increase the vigor with which we start out in the morning,
* maintain and improve our health and well-being,
* make us good-looking and live longer, provided, of course, that we exercise *systematically, vigorously and continually*.

(c) What's the best way to combine aerobic exercises and strength training?

For best results, *alternate* the two major types of exercise to enable your muscles, joints and tendons to recover between intensive workouts.

You can, for instance, do aerobic exercises on Mondays, Wednesdays and Fridays, and reserve Tuesdays and Thursdays for strength training. Saturdays and Sundays would be "natural" for walking or any other enjoyable sports activity.

(d) Do we have to go to a gym to exercise?

Not at all. We can choose from a variety of indoor and outdoor activities. Physically demanding work or household chores are two of them. But best health outcomes are achieved with sports and games involving *systematic* physical activity and exertion.

29. Exercise vigorously enough to make it worthwhile

While some individuals work out too hard (thus risking burnout or injury), most of us are not exerting ourselves sufficiently to get the full benefit of our efforts.

> *To make exercising worthwhile, we should engage in 30 to 60 minutes of moderate physical activity three to six times per week.*

You can choose from the following three ways of determining your age- and fitness-appropriate intensity levels.

(1) TARGET-HEART-RATE METHOD

To use this approach, first calculate your Maximum Heart Rate (MHR).

Begin by subtracting your age from 220. For a 20-year-old individual, for example, the MHR would be 220 minus 20, which equals 200.

Then *take 50 to 70% of the MHR to arrive at the recommended moderate heart-rate range.* For the 20-year old, the range is 100 to 140 heart beats (50 to 70% of the MHR of 200). Other ranges, *for age 40*: 90 to 126; *for age 60*: 80 to 112; *for age 80*: 70 to 98.

Obviously, this method is *based only on age*, not on the individual's fitness.

(2) RATE-OF-PERCEIVED-EXERTION (RPE) METHOD

This method is based on how tired the individual feels.

Someone who is at rest rates a 0. For maximum effort, the rate is 10.

For moderate intensity, the individual should aim for the 4- to 6- level, which is defined as an effort that is between "somewhat hard" and "hard." This range *depends solely on the individual's fitness level*.

(3) TALK-TEST METHOD

Here, moderate exercise is defined as one in which the individual can answer a question but can't carry on a conversation.

Your workout is *too hard* if you have to take a breath between every one of your words, and you're *not exerting yourself enough* if you can sing several phrases of a song without breathing hard.

(4) FACTORING IN YOUR FITNESS LEVEL

The above range of 50-60% of the Maximum Heart Rate (MHR) is applicable at the beginner/low-fitness level.

For someone of *average fitness*, the recommended Target Heart Rate moves up to 60-75%. *This is also the rate that needs to be maintained to lose body fat.* At *high fitness* levels, the target rate is 75-80% of the MHR.

IS MORE BETTER?

You can save yourself lots of pain and aggravation, and will greatly improve the chances of keeping your physical fitness program going, if you heed the following advice:

> *Striving to achieve record*
> *performance may give you a sense*
> *of satisfaction, pride and power.*
>
> *But it will hardly improve your*
> *general health, nor will it improve*
> *your energy. And it will increase*
> *the risk of injury of joints,*
> *ligaments and muscles.*

30. Exercise the right way from the start

Exercise can work wonders for your sleep, energy and mood, or a complete waste of time. It can even endanger your health or life. It's up to you. For your well-being, please keep this in mind:

(1) CONSULT YOUR PHYSICIAN before starting any new exercise routine.

Invalidating previous beliefs, Dr. Jeremy N. Morris and and other pioneering medical practitioners proved beyond a doubt that even heart-attack patients can prolong their lives with carefully monitored exercise programs.

But patients with certain conditions or taking certain types of medications may be ill advised to exercise.

(2) HAVE A COACH or other certified instructor (for instance at a YMCA or health club) get you started to avoid dangerous or useless practices, and to help you to get the most out of the time and effort you invest.

> *Because of lack of know-how, most*
> *individuals don't benefit nearly enough*
> *from their exercise routines.*

(3) GET ADDITIONAL INFORMATION. Even the best coaches and fitness instructors can't possibly know everything about sports and exercising. Moreover, the know-how about best physical-fitness practices keeps evolving. So check reliable information sources from time to time.

31. Tap into trustworthy information sources

The Internet abounds with good (and bad!) information. Finding the right information can be tedious and time-consuming. Here are some worthwhile leads:

MEDLINE PLUS, a service of the U.S. National Library of Medicine and the National Institutes of Health at: *nlm.nih.gov/medlineplus/print/exerciseandphysicalfitness.html* is a superb gateway to much of the Internet's best *free* information on exercising You're likely to find the answers to your questions here, but this can be time-consuming.

DR. SIMON'S BOOK: If you are looking for a shortcut to a <u>very</u> basic physical fitness program, your search is over. *The*

No-Sweat Exercise Plan: Lose Weight, Get Healthy and Live Longer, by Dr. Harvey Simon (published as a *Harvard School Medical Guide* paperback book for $16.95 in December of 2006) may be your best bet. Describing cardio, strength, flexibility and stretching exercises based on solid scientific research, it is an easy-to-read *initiation* into the world of fitness for individuals whose goal is good health and well-being rather than high performance.

"DOCTOR GOOGLE:" Use *Google and other search engines* to access information on specific sports (such as running, swimming, aerobic dancing, etc.).

32. Stick to your exercise program

Even more important than selecting the *exactly* right exercise program is to *adhere* to it.

> *Perseverance is the main key to the*
> *success of any exercise regimen.*

The majority of individuals embarking on fitness programs abandon them in less than six weeks. They "recycle" their good intentions again and again, and never reap the advantages they are seeking. The better life they are aspiring to slips away from them year after year.

To avoid this all-too-common "fate," you may want to consider the following guidelines:

(a) DECIDE AND COMMIT. Take this all-important first "mental" step right now now:

> *Resolve to make exercising just*
> *as non-negotiable as washing*
> *yourself and cleaning your*
> *teeth.*

The return on the time and effort invested in consistent, systematic exercise is sky-high.

(b) KEEP YOUR MIND FOCUSED ON THE POSITIVES. Remind yourself often of the *advantages* you'll gain, such as:
* boosts in energy and happiness,
* radiant health and good looks,
* more fun,
* more and better sex,
* improved performance at work, in sports and every other aspect that contributes to your success.

Don't dwell on "negatives" such as having to give up television-watching time. This is a small price to pay for the huge benefits you'll reap.

(c) BE REALISTIC. Don't try to make overly sweeping lifestyle changes. You may not manage to go to the gym three times a week. But perhaps you can at least fit 30 minutes of walking, or 20 minutes of calisthenics or weight lifting, into every weekday.

(d) DON'T MAKE ANY EXCUSES: ANY TIME'S OK! There's no clear advantage to exercising at any particular time of day. So get going whenever you can or prefer.

If, for instance, you're a "morning person," work out before breakfast. If necessary or preferred, do it during your lunch hour or in the evening.

> *But never exercise within two hours*
> *after a substantial meal, or two hours*
> *before your bedtime.*

(e) SELECT CAREFULLY. Pick your activities with great care:
* Read up on sports, health facilities, exercise programs, etc.
* Find out from friends what they prefer and why.
* Discuss your preferences with your primary care physician.
* Visit spas and health clubs, and take them up on their free-trial offers. Try out their facilities, programs and trainers.
* To be, and remain, motivated, choose what you like best and fits best into your way of life.

> *The better you choose your fitness*
> *program, the easier it will be for*
> *you to make it a permanent part of*
> *your life.*

(f) START SLOWLY. Begin activities modestly—the more modestly the better. Intensify them *very* slowly, gradually and in line with your physical condition.
* Start, for instance, with a few minutes of leisurely, then progressively brisk, and longer, daily walks.
* Later, phase in aerobic exercises and weight lifting.
* Again later, perhaps join a gym and sign up for increasingly demanding group fitness classes.

The less hurriedly you proceed, the more likely you will persevere.

(g) MAKE FIRM COMMITMENTS to your choices. Confirm them to yourself in writing. Post them on "stickies," and place these on your bathroom mirror, computer screen, etc.

(h) PLAN AHEAD: Decide on specific fitness (and other!) goals every night for the following day.

(i) SCHEDULE YOUR WORKOUTS in your calendar, planner, appointment book or computer log for additional reinforcement. Also, share your decisions with friends, colleagues and others who care for you.

(j) MAINTAIN A LOG of your physical activities to keep track of your commitment, perseverance and performance gains.

(k) HAVE FUN. Listen to uplifting music or motivational audio tapes if possible. Vary your routines, your jogging routes, etc. Team up with cheerful colleagues and friends when you jog, go to gym class, etc.

(l) REWARD YOURSELF. After good workouts, do something you like—but not eating a 940-calorie Big Mac Value Meal!

F. Chewing your way to fame, fortune and world-class athletic performance, and other dinnertime habits favoring blissful sleep

33. Finish dinner three hours before bedtime

Grandma said we shouldn't go to sleep "on a full stomach." She was right, of course.

Falling and staying asleep with a bloated, growling or rebellious belly is difficult. Whatever sleep we may get will be shallow—not nearly deep enough.

> *An overloaded digestive tract*
> *prevents us from entering into*
> *the nightly Deep Sleep phases*
> *(Stage-4 Sleep) of each of our*
> *typically five nightly sleep cycles.*

At the very least, digestive overload will prevent us from getting enough Deep Sleep. This is undesirable because Phase-4 Sleep is the one during which most of the nocturnal overhaul of our bodies and minds take place.

Consequently, we won't fully recover from the demands made upon us during our waking hours. We will wake up groggy and fatigued, and this is hardly a promising start of a new day.

Translated into more specific, practical advice, Grandma's wisdom means that *we should eat early.*

Young persons with perfect digestion may be alright if they finish dinner at least *two* hours before "hitting the sack."

> *But everybody else—particularly*
> *older persons—should leave the*
> *dinner table three hours before*
> *bedtime.*

If we go to sleep, for instance, at 11:00 p.m., we should *finish* the last meal of the day by 8:00. Patients with hernia-related heartburn should end their last meals of the day four to five hours before bedtime.

To recapitulate, if we end dinner early, much of the body's digestive work is done when we go to bed.

> *Consequently, more blood is*
> *available for nighttime reinvig-*
> *oration.*
>
> *We multiply our chances*
> *of waking up fully refreshed*
> *and ready to "get going."*

In addition, *we benefit in other important ways* from starting out with more stamina on the "day after," such as:

(a) BETTER MOOD. When we're well rested, we have more of a can-do attitude, are more optimistic, more confident of our abilities and happier than when we're tired.

(b) SHARPER THINKING. During Deep Sleep, the brain consolidates the huge number of impressions it receives during the day. This improves our ability to think, remember, speak, write and reason.

(c) BETTER RELATIONSHIPS. When we are well rested, we are more charismatic, more attuned to the needs of others, calmer in the face of controversy, and more forgiving.

(d) MORE SUCCESS IN BUSINESS. Having more energy is highly correlated with ambition, goal-setting, drive, initiative, hard work, and work of superior quality.

(e) BETTER HEALTH: When we start our days with lots of energy, we are less in need of fighting fatigue with donuts, café-lattes, energy bars, cookies, candy, sugary beverages, energy drinks, caffeine tablets and other short-term "pepper-uppers" that make us obese and/or jittery, and cause us to crave more of the same "bad stuff" soon afterwards.

34. Cut fluids early

This is a "no-brainer." To reduce nighttime bathroom trips, we are smart to heed this advice:

> *Make approximately 8:00 p.m. the*
> *cut-off time for drinking liquids.*

To be avoided more than any other beverages in the evening are alcohol, coffee (including decaf), tea and soda.

As *diuretics*, they remove water from the body by stimulating urination, thus making us thirsty sooner.

35. Lighten up your dinners

Just as important as finishing dinner early is to make them easy to digest. Here's what is particularly worth paying attention to.

EAT LESS. Two-thirds of the U. S. population are overweight or even obese, and our "super-sizing problem" keeps growing at an alarming rate. Most of us should reduce our overall food and beverage intake.

SWITCH BREAKFAST AND DINNER AROUND. To facilitate sound, refreshing sleep, we should make breakfast our biggest and dinner our smallest meal. There's a lot of wisdom in the time-honored recommendation to ...

> *Eat breakfast like a king,*
> *lunch like a prince, and*
> *dinner like a pauper.*

YES, WE CAN HAVE DINNER IN THE MORNING! Because we're usually hard-pressed for time early in the day, having the big meal in the morning may appear to be impractical.

But it's really "no big deal." If we follow the recommendations outlined throughout this book, we can easily get out of bed earlier and have enough time for a bigger breakfast.

OTHER TIME-SAVERS: We can, in addition, save time in the morning by *getting ready the night before*, such as by:
• having the coffee machine ready to be flicked on,
• laying out the clothes we want to wear,
• preparing our breakfast foods, and keeping them accessible in the refrigerator overnight, and

• having our wallets, packed purses or briefcases, keys, outer-wear, umbrellas, etc., handy in a convenient place by the door.

36. Avoid hard-to-digest food

So as not to interfere with sound sleep, it's important for us to stay away from anything that's hard to assimilate.

Particularly difficult to digest—and bad for our health—are *fried foods, full-fat aged cheeses* (such as Camembert, Brie, etc.) as well as *desserts* and other foods that are loaded with trans- and saturated fats.

Although healthy, some other types are no-no's at dinnertime because they place a *heavy load* on the digestive system as well.

This category includes *onions, beans, cabbage, broccoli and other cruciferous vegetables.*

With regard to *spices*, pro's and con's need to be considered case-by-case.

PROS: Spices contribute to the *pleasure of eating* by making certain foods tastier. They can also be rich in antioxidants and have anti-inflammatory and other beneficial health effects.

Some of them (such as cinnamon, ginger and turmeric) can *aid digestion* and, thus, *make sleep more invigorating.*

CONS: Other spices, or spices consumed in excessive quantities, can *prevent Deep Sleep.*

*My advice is to experiment to find
out which spices are good for you
personally.*

LIMIT VARIETY. The more *different types of food* are combined in your dinner, the longer they will take to digest. A prime example of sabotaging one's sleep in a delightful way would be dining at a buffet restaurant with an irresistible selection of food.

37. Cultivate the art of chewing well (and learn how to become rich and famous doing it)

Mother was right, again, when she admonished us to chew our food well. *Masticating our dinners thoroughly* is at least as important for the enjoyment of invigorating sleep as dining early enough and avoiding hard-to-digest food.

With good chewing habits, we can *reduce or eliminate:*
* *delayed, shallow and interrupted sleep,*
* *common digestive problems* such as burping, gas and bloating, as well as
* *more serious health issues* such as Candida or other types of bacterial overgrowth, heartburn, acid reflux, digestive cramps and irritable bowel syndrome.

Chewing well is not a new idea. But with a view to our present obesity epidemic, it is timely to remind ourselves of the principles championed in the Victorian Age by the American businessman-turned-nutrition-guru *Horace Fletche*r (1849 -1919).

He admonished his contemporaries to pay attention to how they chew their food.

I'll explain in a moment what this has to do with obesity and becoming rich.

During most of his life, *Fletcher suffered from debilitating indigestion and obesity.* Afraid of impending death, he started to seek a solution to his increasing health problems when he was 46 years old.

Through trial and error, he developed a set of *nutritional guidelines* that gradually restored his health and enabled him to become a *competitive athlete of extraordinary endurance* at a mature age.

He soon taught millions of followers around the world health-promoting principles such as:
* *Eat only when you're genuinely hungry.*
* *Take three breaths before eating, and express your gratitude for nature's bounty before you start your meal.*
* *Select only foods that your appetite is craving.* (Important: in Fletcher's time, most of the foods available to consumers were still natural, unprocessed and unadulterated.)
* *Put only small quantities into your mouth.*
* *Drink little or not at all with meals, and never wash food down with beverages.*
* *Eat slowly.* Put your knives and forks down every time after having swallowed.
* *Eat only until you're satisfied — not full.*

> *But the core of his teachings — the*
> *advice that made him healthy, rich*
> *and famous — is that we chew each*

> *small mouthful of food 32 times*
> *("once for each of the teeth in our*
> *mouths").*

More specifically, he recommended that we *caress the texture of the food with our tongues* and allow our taste buds to *savor the rich flavors* of every bite until all taste remnants have been extracted.

> *This, he argued, will give our*
> *minds enough time to tell our*
> *stomachs that we've had enough,*
> *and will keep us slim.*

Fletcher promoted his nutritional doctrine (called *"Fletcherism"*) relentlessly through his writings and speaking engagements around the world.

He became a multi-millionaire at a time when the dollar was worth a lot more than today.

He also earned kudos for his massive contributions to public health from world-class universities as well as global opinion leaders in politics, health, medicine, philosophy, literature and business.

He was consulted by people of renown like Upton Sinclair and John D. Rockefeller, and entertained dignitaries like Henry James and Mark Twain at his palazzo in Venice.

When he died of a heart attack at age 69 in 1919, his fame in the field of nutrition was being eclipsed by a new, no less revolutionary dieting movement—the one spearheaded by two other brilliant Americans, Irving Fisher and Eugene Lyman Fisk: *counting calories*.

....

Hugo Tschudin's personal perspective

When I was a pre-teen living in Switzerland, my family occasionally entertained one of my father's best friends at Sunday dinners.

As an openly "Fletcherizing" individual, *our guest chewed every mouthful 32 times* at the super-efficient speed of about one hundred chops per minute (no kidding!). This was recommended, he said, by nutrition expert Horace Fletcher.

My brother and I were in awe of this spectacle.

More than six decades after these unforgettable meals, and a few days before I wrote the first draft of this book, I read Mr. Fletcher's writings and decided to give his approach a chance to prove itself in *my* life.

Adding to my motivation was the fact that I had just gained five pounds within one week and was plagued by bothersome stomach rumblings.

Impressed by Mr. Fletcher's insistence on eating only when we are not merely stressed but *really* hungry, I skipped breakfast for a day. I didn't even want to "eat like a pauper!" I felt somewhat full anyway—so why should I have breakfast at all?

Should I eat out of habit, or because nutrition gurus like Keith (W.K.) Kellogg had preached that skipping breakfast is a bad idea and eating his flaked cereals a good one?

My decision to forego breakfast proved to be surprisingly beneficial. Rather than being tired by working "on an empty stomach," I felt great and wrote Mr. Fletcher's "story" (the one you're reading here) in record time.

Continuing to feel no need to eat, I skipped lunch as well, and worked out at the health club after having eaten only a few whole-wheat crackers.

From then on, I reduced the quantity and types of food consumed, thus following Mr. Fletcher's advice. Consequently, *I easily lost the five pounds I had gained,* and have kept them off ever since (knock on wood!).

Do I chew 32 times? No! I vary the number of "chops" depending on the texture of the food. In line with Fletcher's reasoning, I am chewing longer overall than ever before. I keep chewing until the food is completely liquefied and there's no more taste to be extracted from it.

Guess what: I feel better than before my re-discovery of "the GREAT MASTICATOR.

....

Many of us gobble down snacks or entire meals mindlessly while watching television. Or we eat as if we were out to establish a new *Guinness-speed-eating record.* Sooner or later, we will pay a heavy price for such destructive habits.

If we take more time for deliberate chewing, our DIGESTION WILL IMPROVE DRAMATICALLY FOR SEVERAL REASONS.

(1) INCREASED FOOD SURFACE. The mechanical breakdown into small particles increases the food's exposure to saliva.

(2) MORE "ENZYME POWER." The longer we chew, the *more quickly and efficiently* the enzymes in the saliva will go to work on the food while it's still in the mouth. This is especially important for carbohydrates and fat. It reduces the digestive work of the stomach and intestines.

(3) BETTER PREPARATION FOR WHAT'S COMING. In the stomach, chewing stimulates the production of hydrochloric acid (essential especially for breaking down protein). And in the small intestines, it triggers the secretion of other essential enzymes.

(4) BETTER PROTECTION AGAINST OBESITY. The brain is slow in registering satiety. This has important implications for individuals who want to keep their weight down.

The longer we chew our food, the less we have to consume until the brain senses that we have had enough.

Thus, "Fletcherism" reduces the danger of eating too much food and becoming obese.

38. Don't go to bed half-starved

Earlier (above, No. 33), we warned against eating dinner late (such as after 8 o'clock).

> *But equally problematic is*
> *eating too early.*

If you eat very early (such as because of special scheduling requirements while traveling, or to benefit from a restaurant's early-bird dinner bargain), it's advisable to consume a *small pre-bed snack*.

Otherwise, low nutrient levels in the blood will cause the feeding center of the hypothalamus to make you raid the refrigerator and eat during the night.

> *If we don't give in to the*
> *craving, hunger can keep*
> *us awake all night.*

While this link between hunger and wakefulness is proven beyond a doubt, it's far less certain of WHAT TYPE OF FOOD a pre-bed snack should ideally consist. There are three different schools of thought.

(1) PROTEINS: Some experts recommend tryptophan-rich proteins (such as small quantities of unsweetened yogurt, or a few slices of turkey meat), because they relax the central nervous system. But this view appears to be based more on folklore than on solid scientific evidence because the quantities of tryptophan contained in such snacks are minor.

(2) CARBOHYDRATES: Others prefer carbs such as a few whole-wheat crackers or a small slice of whole-grain bread, arguing that carbohydrate-induced highs are soon followed by calmer moods. Bananas offer an additional advantage; their high level of magnesium makes it easier to relax.

(3) COMBINATIONS: Again others advocate commingling— such as eating crackers with either some chicken meat or sliced turkey, or drinking warm, honey-sweetened milk.

WHAT'S RIGHT FOR YOU? The answer depends on the timing and quantity of your snack, and perhaps also your "nutritional type." So my best recommendation may again be that you *experiment* to find out what's *best for you.*

> *More importantly, we should not*
> *let pre-bedtime snacking degenerate*
> *into mindless nightly eating binges.*

Regardless of our choice of pre-bed snacks, we should always remember to *brush our teeth* afterwards to prevent tooth decay.

39. Think twice before wetting your whistle with an alcoholic "nightcap"

Alcohol is not only consumed during "happy hour" after work, but also at dinnertime and afterwards (in which case it's commonly referred to as a "nightcap").

Because we're dealing with the same types of substances, the information provided in connection with the "happy hour" (above, No. 23) also applies here—in connection with "nightcaps."

As mentioned, alcoholic beverages initially enhance our mood and *facilitate falling asleep*. But the sleep they induce is short, fitful, shallow, and *usually followed by hangovers*.

In our search for *better alternatives* we may again want to take a look at Grandma's box of magic tricks. Among them are:
* *warm, soothing milk* (containing mildly sedative tryptophan—but so little that its potential effectiveness appears to be based mostly on the placebo effect),
* *chamomile tea* (prepared from the flower of this herb), and
* *valerian* (in powder capsules or extract drops prepared from the plant's roots).

Who cares that Grandma's remarkable success as a healer may be rooted at least in part in the placebo effect and the power of gentle persuasion!

G. Futile and beneficial pre-bed practices

40. Put left-over anger, worries or other negative baggage to rest

Now, in the evening, is the time to come to terms with *harmful emotions* that have not been properly dealt with earlier in the day.

We can't permit them to mar our leisure-time. It would be even worse to take them to bed with us.

> *One good way to solve this problem is JOURNALING. Write down, every evening, whatever may still be troubling your mind, to unburden it.*

Add your thoughts on how you might *solve* the problems.

Also, outline *simple plans* (with perhaps three or four action steps each) on how to deal with every one of them either immediately or at a more suitable time.

Another good approach is the *TWO-COLUMN METHOD*. Take a piece of paper and draw a vertical line through the middle.

On the left side, write down your *concerns* one by one. *To their right,* jot down the *solutions* that come to mind, or what you intend to do to find solutions later, when it's more convenient.

41. Steer clear of anything that might upset you

Stay away from experiences and activities that may stimulate, upset or worry you, such as:
• *TV programs* that get the adrenaline going: newscasts, game and adventure shows, horror movies, hyped-up commercials, etc.
• competitive board as well as video and other *games,*
• family-problem-solving and other *spirited discussions,*
• *Internet surfing,*
• job-related *work,*
• *payments* of bills, or efforts to balance the budget, etc.

42. Switch to a twilight setting

> *One of the most important ways to prepare yourself for sleep is to darken your room.*

When the retina on the inner surface of our eyes ceases to perceive light, our biological clocks spring into action.

They signal the brain that it's time to get ready to sleep by causing the pineal gland to *release melatonin into the blood stream.*

Melatonin is a hormone that regulates the circadian rhythm.

"Circadian" is derived from "circa" (Latin for "around") and "dies" (Latin for "day"), thus meaning "around 24 hours."
So the circadian rhythm is the approximately-24-hour cycle of sleep and wakefulness.

> *When light fades away, melatonin is se-*
> *creted by the brain's pineal gland, which*
> *makes us drowsy and induces sleep.*

And when daylight returns, the flow of melatonin dries up, which promotes wakefulness.

Here is how you can get this melatonin-controlled calming process under way:
* *Dim the lights around you.*
* Draw black-out curtains to insulate yourself from outside light.
* For reading, use a reading lamp at the lowest suitable setting.
* End your exposure to light from large TV screens and computer monitors.
* Have low-voltage night lights in place to guide your steps.
* Use eye shades if it's impractical to darken your room.

> *Melatonin is widely available as a*
> *prescription-free food supplement*
> *in the United States.*

In addition to being a sleep aid, it's also a powerful antioxidant. But it can have some (mostly minor) undesirable effects (especially drug interactions). For details, see No. 68 below.

43. Unwind with quiet "me-time"

> *Develop a pre-bedtime rite as a*
> *cue for your mind to settle down*
> *and get ready to fall asleep.*

Here are a few *examples* of such rituals:
* *Read* something soothing such as a book of meditations, or something boring such as a chemistry textbook.
* *Meditate* or pray.
* Use *affirmations* such as:
  >> *"I'm in harmony with life."*
  >> *"Peace is within me."*
  >>*"I'm relaxing ... relaxing ... relaxing ..."*
* Do *breathing* and Progressive Relaxation Exercises.
* *Visualize* bucolic, lakeside or other tranquil landscapes.
* *Listen to soft music* or CD's with soothing messages or sounds, such as gently rolling ocean waves, or chirping insects at dusk.

44. Cool off your bedroom

Falling asleep is easier if we lower our bedroom temperatures before going to bed.

> *Set the thermostat between 60 and 70*
> *degrees F (16 to 21 degrees C), or*
> *generate a cooling breeze with a fan.*

To understand why cooling your bedroom makes falling asleep easier, you must know that our body temperature varies by about 2 degrees F (about 1 degree C) during a 24-hour period, and that it is lower when we're asleep than during our waking hours.

> *Lowering our body temperature*
> *to the sleep level by cooling the*

> *bedroom makes us tired and*
> *drowsy when the night approaches.*

Sleeping in a cool (but not freezing) bedroom has another beneficial effect. It makes our night rest more invigorating by inducing more *Deep Sleep.*

For most inhabitants of temperate climates, the ideal temperature for Deep Sleep is in the 60-to-70-degree range. (My personal preference is 78 degrees.)

> *It's eminently worth experimenting*
> *to find out which temperature is*
> *best for you.*

Lowering your bedroom temperature is particularly important under two circumstances: in steamy hot summer nights, and in winter if the bedroom is overheated.

45. Take a hot or warm bath or shower

To make falling asleep easier, also consider what only *appears* to be counterproductive: raising your body temperature by taking a hot (or warm) bath or shower before bedtime.

The reason for this is that ...

> *When we COOL OFF late in the*
> *evening, after having been warmed*
> *up, we become increasingly tired*
> *and sleepy.*

This approach has the same sleep-inducing cooling effect as lowering the temperature of your bedroom as mentioned above. For best outcomes, the bath or shower should be taken about 90 minutes prior to bedtime.

But for some individuals, shorter time intervals may be more effective.

For others, baths or showers taken *at any time* will be counterproductive, making it harder rather than easier to enter the Land of Nod later on.

> *Again, it's worth experiment-*
> *ting to find out what's best for*
> *you.*

Bathing or showering is particularly beneficial for sedentary persons. They are neither tired enough from physical activity, nor can they benefit from sufficiently big drops in body temperature.

There are several ways to make baths even more relaxing:
• Dim the lights.
• Listen to soft background music.
• Use a rolled-up towel or waterproof pillow to support your neck and head.
• Gently stretch, and then relax, your limbs.
• Use Progressive Relaxation, one muscle group at a time.
• While you continue soaking, read a page or two from a relaxing book that puts your mind at ease.

Hot water strips the skin of its natural oils. These may have to be replaced with skin lotions (preferably products that are free of unnecessary artificial preservatives and fragrances).

To bring about the desired cooling effect without taking a bath or shower, some people are reported to *chill their pillows in their refrigerators* for a few minutes.

46. Don't go to bed until you're VERY tired

Going to bed at the same time every day appears to make a lot of sense, and is held in high regard not only by disciplined, solid citizens but also by scores of misinformed writers of articles in the mass media who copy from each other.

But it's a bad mistake. It's unrealistic and rarely practical. Above all, it *can cause sleepers to toss and turn in bed for hours.* They can become more and more worried about their perceived inability to get enough sleep.

> *One of the mast important keys to sleeping soundly is NOT turning in at a certain predetermined time, and NOT when you're just SOMEWHAT TIRED, but waiting until you're TOTALLY DRAINED and drowsy.*

Your ability to think and act should be severely impaired.

> *The time when you're sleepy and ready for bed varies from individual to individual and from day to day.*

It depends on the sleep you had the night before, the work you performed, the stress you were under, the exercises you did, the coffee you drank, the sunshine you got, etc.

There's something to be said in favor of regularity, though. Setting boundaries *is* important. Going to bed whenever you are very tired, and rising whenever you happen to wake up, hinders the development of *efficient sleep patterns,* wastes time and is incompatible with society's need to synchronize activities.

So what's the best way out of this dilemma? The best advice offered by *up-to-date* sleep experts is:

> *GO TO BED whenever you're very tired, but GET UP at the same predetermined time every day.*

If you're still tired when it's time to get out of bed, *get up anyway.* To compensate for lost sleep, you'll be ready to go to bed earlier at the end of the day. Thus, you'll catch up with your need for sleep without changing your daily sleep *starting point.*

47. Get relief

> *Go to the bathroom before retiring.*

It's difficult to sleep with a full bladder. Urinating once a night is considered by many medical professionals to be normal.

But "having to go" *more than once every night* is a somewhat more serious condition. Called *NOCTURIA,* it usually results in tiresome sleep deficits.

Nocturia—not to be confused with *ENURESIS* (bedwetting)— plagued almost two thirds of adults between the ages of 55 and 84 who responded to a National Sleep Foundation poll taken in 2003.

The elderly are most at risk because, as we advance in age, our bodies produce less of an antidiuretic hormone (a chemical messenger that slows down the production of urine at night).

> *Measures to stop or at least*
> *minimize nocturia and enuresis*
> *include stopping the intake of*
> *fluids at least two hours—and*
> *preferably three—before bed-*
> *time.*

If this doesn't help, it's advisable to seek the help of your primary care physician who may, in turn, refer you to a sleep or other specialist, or to a sleep laboratory, for testing.

Thanks to the availability of advanced tests and medications, nocturia and enuresis sufferers have excellent chances of overcoming these energy-sapping conditions with the support of competent medical professionals.

H. Romantic and other actions to prepare for the most satisfying and refreshing sleep ever

48. Invite romance

Now comes the fun part for couples!
- *Make up.*
- *Massage each other.*
- *Cuddle.*
- *Kiss.*
- *Embrace.*
- *Make love.*

But watch out, ladies and gentlemen: this is controversial!

For many—especially men—the combination of physical and emotional communication with a "significant other" is *one of nature's most satisfying sleep aids.* BUT:

> *Women often complain that their*
> *lovers fall asleep long before they*
> *(the women) are satisfied.*

One lady blogger opined that men are selfish and too lazy to meet women's needs once they had *their* orgasms.

One excuse for men's premature flabbiness is that sex is usually more exhausting for them than for women. More plausible is another explanation—the one that ...

> *During ejaculation, oxytocin and*
> *vasopressin are released into the*

*men's bloodstream, and that these
natural chemicals cause sleepiness.*

So if men start snoring while women are still yearning for more, they may merely surrender to biochemical forces. But is this a good-enough argument?

Incidentally, withholding their charms to retaliate for the alleged indifference of male companions may not be a wise policy for women because oxytocin and vasopressin also have *social attachment (emotional bonding) effects.*

What are devoted men to do to make their women happy?
* One possibility is to *elongate foreplay*. While men can go from arousal to orgasm in as few as three minutes, some women need in excess of twenty minutes to get theirs.
* Another bliss-promoting tip for men is to *take deep breaths* when they approach their orgasms to enable themselves to stay awake and "carry on" (Good Luck!--the proof reader).

Anyway, with mutual understanding and respect, physical intimacy can be *nature's greatest prelude to invigorating sleep.*

49. Avoid pain in the neck

Once you're resting in bed, make sure you avoid pain in the neck.

Shore up your pillow so it cradles your head in a comfortable position and gives your neck the support it needs to avoid muscle strain.

Shun the *face-down position* to prevent neck and back strain as well as pressure on the stomach.

> *Sleep on your side. Or position*
> *yourself on your back, with your*
> *arms by your side.*

Put a second pillow under your top leg (if you sleep on your side) or under your knees (if you sleep on your back). Adjust your pillows and your position to relieve potential pressure points.

Now make just one more adjustment. Loosen and flatten ("un-wrinkle") any confining clothing.

This may be unnecessary if you use slippery silk sleepwear. If desired for comfort, sleep in the nude if your bedroom temperature permits.

Resting on a *good mattress in good condition* is another "must." This is obvious but often overlooked because their deterioration is very gradual.

50. Become a drifter

> *When you're "all set," don't make*
> *any effort to fall asleep.*

Don't try to *will* yourself to sleep

Don't even *think* about sleeping. Thinking about it is the worst course of action. It has the exact opposite effect. It *keeps* you thinking.

Instead, just let yourself go. Become a drifter!

Permit yourself to nod off effortlessly.

"Sink" into your mattress in a relaxed way, and simply accept somnolence as one of nature's great blessings. Sleep in peace!

....

What if you're not done?

If you have come this far, congratulations are in order. This could be the end of your journey to divine sleep—assuming, of course, that you have taken the previous recommendations to heart.

But what if you are still not getting the sleep you need to get up happily and with energy to spare on the following day?

Then try the subsequent proven strategies, especially the one that follows.

....

51. Don't ever lose sleep over losing sleep

Be patient.

Some of us can fall asleep almost immediately. But it is far more likely for the transition to slumber to take about 15 minutes or even somewhat longer.

So take it easy. Relax. Stay calm.

Don't worry even if it takes you more time than usual to lose yourself in slumber.

> *You'll function surprisingly well*
> *on the day after a sleepless night —*
> *provided you don't fret about it.*

The fear of failure on the following day is usually vastly exaggerated. But even if it isn't, worrying about it won't make falling asleep easier.

In fact, the opposite is true. *The longer and the more deeply you worry* about your perceived inability to fall asleep, the more your *fear will become part of your subconscious mind,* and the more you risk developing *chronic insomnia.*

52. Relegate your fears, anger or other negative emotions to a "Worry Pad"

When you're in bed it's not a good time to fret or be upset about anything.

A *Worry Pad* and a writing instrument placed on your night table can be used with great success to escape from the tyranny of upsetting emotions.

> *Write down the concerns that keep*
> *racing through your mind, and*
> *promise yourself to get back to*
> *them on the following day.*

Worries, fears and anger *often disappear overnight.*

Helpful ideas will sooner or later come to our rescue. These inspirations are often so good that we are far better off than before we perceived the bothersome problems.

53. Don't count sheep, nor practice "thought suppression"

Finally, it turns out that Grandma was *not* infallible.

Imagining sheep and silently counting them, one by one, while they're jumping over a fence, was supposed to make one's mind focus on one easy task to the exclusion of all other thoughts. But it proved to be an *ineffective mental exercise* for lulling oneself to sleep.

In a *study conducted at England's Oxford University*, the sleeping patterns of 50 insomniacs divided into four groups were observed:
- GROUP A, the control group, was left to fall asleep as usual (without having been given any instructions).
- GROUP B was asked to "count sheep."
- GROUP C was told to use "thought suppression" (meaning that they should block out any troubling thoughts as soon as they occurred).
- GROUP D was directed to imagine a tranquil scene such as a beach or a peaceful waterfall.

The results were enlightening.

- GROUP B, *the "sheep counters,"* took a little longer to nod off than the control group (A). Thus, counting sheep proved to be *ineffective* and even slightly counterproductive.

Some experts speculated that this method was disappointing because it was *boring* and the sleepers couldn't keep it up. Others thought that seeing jumping animals was *too exciting* to have a calming effect. They favored counting *resting* sheep instead.

• GROUP C, *the "thought suppressors,"* were *least successful.* They fell asleep 10 minutes later than the control group. (This agreed with the famous experiment in which participants were instructed *not* to think about *black* polar bears, which made them think *even more* about them.)

• GROUP D, *who imagined tranquil scenes,* were *most successful.* They fell asleep 20 minutes sooner. (More on this strategy will be found under No. 57 below.)

Not timed was another frequently recommended trick. Sleepers were directed to think of something boring to keep bothersome thoughts away.

They were asked to carry out simple *repetitive mathematical operations* such as counting backwards from 200 to zero, or reciting multiples of 3 ("3, 6, 9," etc.). Results were quite satisfactory.

> *But method D—using guided imager was usually far more effective.*

I. Taking the struggle out of nodding off: how to ease yourself into somnolence and—finally—blissful sleep

54. Meditate or pray

More effective than counting sheep or counting backwards from 200 is *meditating on a calming word or phrase, or silently reciting mantras such as:*

- *"Ohm ... ohm ... ohm ... "*
- *"Sleep well ... well ... well ..."*
- *"Mind empty ... empty ... empty ..."*
  or simply:
- *"Peace ... peace ... peace ..."*

Religious believers may prefer to seek and find serenity by *opening their hearts and minds to God.* They may, for instance, achieve perfect inner peace by surrendering their fears, worries, struggles and endeavors to the Almighty.

Both meditation and prayer are known to be conducive to sleep by *slowing down our heart rate and breathing*, reducing our blood pressure and relaxing our muscles. Thus, they mimic the way we function in our sleep.

55. Take deep, slow belly breaths

If, by now, you *still* need to do more to fall asleep, it's time to focus on the way you breathe.

Lying on your back, inhale deeply for three slow counts (counting "twenty-one, twenty-two, twenty-three").

Start inhaling into the *bottom* part of your lungs so that your belly and diaphragm get extended.

Then exhale for three equally slow counts. Do this for about five minutes.

For more details, please return to No. 16, part (a).

56. Practice Progressive Muscle Relaxation (PMR)

One step up from breathing techniques is Progressive Muscle Relaxation, a more elaborate stress management method.

Developed by *Dr. Edmund Jacobson,* it can be highly effective. It's more difficult to master but worth the extra effort.

> *When practiced in bed, this method*
> *usually leads seamlessly into sleep.*
> *This makes it one of the best weapons*
> *against insomnia.*

PMR is also an outstanding daytime stress-reduction technique. It's often favored by persons who feel "uptight" or "tense" (terms that are indicative of their links to *muscle stress*).

It's effective in relieving tension headaches, muscle spasms, backaches, tightness around the eyes, high blood pressure, anxiety and more.

*PMR entails alternatively tightening
and relaxing muscle groups one by one.*

After the muscles are relaxed, they will be more loose and limp than before the tensing. Thanks to the body-mind connection, this will change one's mood.

Individuals using PMR become calmer.

WARNING: PMR should not be used by persons with a history of serious injuries, pulled muscles, muscle spasms, back problems, broken bones or torn ligaments as well as by patients who should not engage in physical activities. The tensing could exacerbate such pre-existing conditions.

....

Progressive Muscle Relaxation in a Nutshell

The recommended procedure is as follows:
* Get comfortable in your bed (or in an armchair in a quiet corner).
* Take three deep abdominal breaths ("belly breaths"). Feel the relief when you exhale slowly.
* Concentrate on one major muscle group at a time (such as first hands, then biceps/triceps, then shoulders, etc.). Tense them progressively for about ten seconds each until they begin to feel uncomfortable. Do so while you inhale, inflating first—and mostly—the bottom part of the lungs.
* Then let the muscles relax and become loose for about 10 to 15 seconds as you exhale, and use an affirmation such as *"It's OK!"* or *"Let go!"* Feel the built-up tension melt, dissolve and flow away.

• Do this tensing-and-releasing routine for all major muscle groups. Also relax your tongue and jaw, as well as your facial muscles.

CALMING EFFECT: The more your relaxation spreads through your body, the more you will calm down. As stated by Dr. Jacobson, *"an anxious mind cannot exist in a relaxed body."*

TIME REQUIRED: Initially, Progressive Muscle Relaxation will take about 20 minutes. But after having gained sufficient experience with it, practitioners can proceed much more quickly.

....

Hugo Tschudin's personal observations

Based on my investigations, *I highly recommend Progressive Muscle Relaxation.* This technique requires an investment of time and effort.

But the benefits of PMR are worth far more than what we put into it—especially for individuals suffering from tension headaches and "knots in the stomach," as well as for those of us who find it difficult to shut off bothersome anxiety, concerns and troubles racing through our minds at bedtime.

Am I using PMR? Frankly: no! In the rare cases when I find it difficult to relax—in and out of bed—I'm using a method that's similar to PMR, the *Autogenic Training.* This method was developed before PMR and presented to the public for the first time in 1927 by the German psychiatrist Johannes Heinrich Schultz.

I was trained in the use of this autosuggestion-based relaxation technique while I was a student in my native country, Switzerland.

Rather than being based on muscle tensing and relaxation (as in PMR), Autogenic Training induces deep relaxation by suggesting that specific muscles or muscle groups *feel heavy and subsequently warm.*

This leads to increased blood flow to the respective muscles accompanied by a trance-like deep relaxation.

This is, in turn, followed by other steps, such as calming one's breathing and heartbeat, as well as meditation and post-hypnotic autosuggestions.

....

How to benefit even more from PMR and Autogenic Training

There's much more to know about PMR and Autogenic Training than what can be made to fit into this book. For further study I recommend the following resource:

- *Guidetopsychology.com/pmr/htm.* This site offers an excellent free description of PMR. It's short but contains enough information for the casual student of PMR.

For more in-depth study, I propose the concurrent use of the following book and CD:
- *The Relaxation and Stress Reduction Workbook* by Martha Davis, Elizabeth Robbins and Matthew McKay. This book contains concise, easy-to-follow descriptions of PMR,

Autogenic Training and other stress-reduction techniques.
It has been called the "bible" in its field.

- *Progressive Relaxation and Autogenic Training* by Carolyn
McManus with music by Stella Benson (harpist). The first
track of this CD guides listeners through PMR, and the
second is their introduction to Autogenic Training.

57. Use the magic of guided imagery to drift off to sleep

This is another superb technique for lulling oneself to sleep. It
can be used either by itself or in combination with the previous three approaches (meditation/prayer, breathing, and
PMR).

> *To use guided imagery, we mentally*
> *conjure up a tranquil place (or a*
> *soothing color like green, light*
> *blue or lavender) to enter into a*
> *relaxed state of mind that makes*
> *us fall asleep.*

This method is effective because of the "wiring" between
body and mind.

It causes the brain to *trigger the release of hormones that act as
gentle tranquilizers.* We respond by falling asleep as if the
tranquilizing scene we are imagining were real.

To remove doubts about the *awesome power of the body/mind
connection,* imagine holding a fresh, juicy lemon in your
hands. "See" its intense yellow color, and "feel" the texture of

its peel. And now imagine yourself slicing it or biting into it with the sour juice squirting out.

Chances are your salivary glands have already swung into action; your guided imagery made you salivate.

Here's the best way to ease yourself into sleep with this technique:

• *Get comfortable* in your bed and close your eyes.

• *Imagine yourself sitting on a blanket or cozy folding chair in one of your favorite peaceful places* such as a secluded beach at dusk. "See" and "hear" the gently breaking waves, "smell" the salty air and "watch" that awe-inspiring sunset. Or, in your "mind's eye," sit down on a bench in a fragrant flower garden, or overlooking a peaceful valley, or whatever soothing setting you may prefer.

• *Now feel how your tension is fading* and your heartbeat slowing down. You are more and more at peace. You simply let yourself go and effortlessly drift off to sleep.

> *In the unlikely case that you are*
> *still awake, you say to yourself:*
> • *"I'm calm and relaxed,"*
> • *"I'm letting go," or*
> • *"I'm drifting off to sleep ...*
> *sleep ... sleep," or*
> • *"Peace ... peace ... peace ..."*

If guided imagery doesn't help you to overcome insomnia at first try, it's good to remind yourself that *practice makes perfect.* It's worth working at it every night until you succeed.

58. Use Guided Imagery also as a daytime self-help tool for the pursuit of any worthwhile goal (including world-class athletic performance)

Practicing Guided Imagery exclusively to imagine ourselves into somnolence is a humongous waste of the extraordinary success potential of this *extraordinarily powerful universal self-help tool.*

> *Guided Imagery can be used to*
> *pave the way to virtually any*
> *worthwhile goal regardless of*
> *its type or magnitude.*

The more we practice it, the more we increase its awesome power in our lives.

Guided Imagery is particularly useful for reaching bold "stretch goals."

Easily the best-known arena of widespread application is the world of *high-performance sports.*

> *There's hardly any top athlete*
> *who's not using guided imagery*
> *to condition him- or herself to*
> *perform at record-breaking levels.*

We can use guided imagery equally well to *reach an almost unlimited array of objectives,* such as to:
• fall asleep,
• overcome fatigue and increase endurance,

- relieve pain,
- boost immunity,
- accelerate healing and overcome illness,
- lose weight,
- quit smoking and conquer drug abuse,
- put an end to "negativity," unhappiness, depression and phobias,
- overcome fear of failure, procrastination, shyness and stage fright,
- win a sports competition, and
- develop enthusiasm, initiative and other desirable personality traits.

When your visualization has induced the desired *relaxed state* of body and mind, you're *ready to use affirmations* depending on your *specific* needs.

IN BED, you may want to visualize yourself as being about to fall asleep (as mentioned earlier).

DURING THE DAY, your visualization may be that you're calming down and becoming more and more relaxed ... or perking up and making headway with your work .... or getting healthier ... or whatever your need may be *at that time.*

Instead of making affirmations right away, visualize yourself first in a relaxing scenery (for better access to the subconscious mind), and then in the state or circumstances you wish to reach.

The more you practice Guided Imagery, the more quickly and intensely you'll be able to conjure up the desired effect.

For more details, please return to the information on affirmations in Nos. 6 to 9 above.

59. Give yourself another chance later

If you're *still* not asleep after about 15 to 30 minutes, don't remain in bed "trying" to sleep (and probably worrying about it). Instead ...

> *Get up! Go to another room. Do*
> *something—anything—that relaxes*
> *you.*

Look out of the window if you live in serene surroundings. Or just relax in a comfortable chair.

Choose from any of the *calming options* we are already familiar with:
* Meditate, or listen to soft music or a soothing CD.
* Use positive affirmations.
* Practice deep-breathing (but with longer-than-usual intervals, to avoid energizing yourself) ... Progressive Muscle Relaxation or Autogenic Training ... or use Guided Imagery (visualizing tranquil, serene scenes)..
* Read a soothing book (in dim light so as not to chase away your melatonin).
* Banish your worries to a Worry Pad, and relegate your thoughts and ideas to your journal.
* Take a warm bath or shower.

Or play solitaire—a card game for one person that was designed to make the player fall asleep.

Whatever you do, be patient.

Your time to yield to the urge to sleep will come.

*Return to bed only when you
can't keep your eyes open any
longer.*

Then you will be more than ready for the blessings of sleep.

60. Make waking up with lots of energy a never-ending passion

If you are waking up refreshed and "raring to go," you're blessed. It's also an indication that you're taking good care of your body and mind and live in harmony with your surroundings.

*If, however, you're starting "on
empty" every morning, this is a
signal for you to examine the way
you live. It tells you that your
lifestyle is in need of a review
and tune-up.*

Whenever this happens, it may be time for you to *return to this book for use as your "lifestyle checklist."* Read it again to identify the strategies from which you deviated.

Mark the ones requiring corrective action. The result will be your *Personal Energy Management Plan.*

Put the Plan's *"action items"* on your agenda or to-do list, and concentrate on each action long enough to turn it into a good, lasting habit.

> *Remaining on the right path*
> *requires constant vigilance, but*
> *is worth a big multiple of the*
> *price you paid for it.*

Staying the course will give you an *abundance of power* to make your journey through life amazingly joyful and rewarding—the way it's meant to be!

J. Forever more energetic, successful and happy

61. Congratulations! Now what?

You've come a long way, dear reader:
* You know that "getting going" in the morning doesn't have to be a struggle for the rest of your life.
* You know that it's in your power to change.
* You know how to energize yourself from the time when you wake up.
* You know how to make getting up the welcome beginning of a glorious day.

> *SO NOW JUST DO IT! Follow the advice, using this book as your inspiration and guide.*

Above all, control your thinking. If you maintain that you will "always wake up tired," you will *indeed* start every day in a state of fatigue.

> *Your subconscious mind is that powerful.*

By this time, you've probably liberated yourself already from the tyranny of self-fulfilling negative expectations and *know*— not only intellectually but also deep-down inside you—that you *can* "perk up" if you follow proven protocols.

Maybe you have already:
* begun an exercise program,

- started to unwind after work,
- changed some of your dining habits,
- adopted better bedtimes,
- made good bedroom improvements,
- learned to put your mind at ease once you're in bed ... etc.

> *Whatever you have done so far*
> *has probably improved the*
> *way you feel not only at the*
> *beginning of your day but also*
> *throughout your waking hours.*

Chances are the *people around you have noticed the differences* and are drawn more to you now. They see a "new you."

You are more energetic, more productive, happier, friendlier, more cheerful and more optimistic. You also look better than when you were fatigued and downcast.

> *When friends and acquaintances*
> *ask you about your transformation,*
> *by all means tell them how great*
> *you feel.*
>
> *Describe the changes that made it*
> *happen. But don't volunteer this*
> *information.*
>
> *Above all, don't criticize their*
> *lifestyles, and be careful not to*
> *"preach."*

They'll come to you for guidance if and when they are ready for it.

But what if you encounter seemingly insurmountable *obstacles* on your way to more energy, greater vitality and a better quality of life?

If this happens to you, don't get discouraged. It happens to all of us, and we can take remedial action. We can succeed!

....

Hugo Tschudin's confession

Here's a good place for me to come clean.

I wrote this book, of course, and Energizing Life is not only my passion but also my mission. It's even the URL of my website (www.EnergizingLife.com).

But this doesn't make me perfect. I'm not always bursting with energy.

I'm not talking about healthy fatigue here (what I propose to call *eufatigue* in analogy to the word *eustress,* which was coined by Hans Selye to denote the healthy, invigorating type of stress).

I welcome eufatigue into my life—the type of fatigue resulting from exercise and other initiatives in order for me to sleep well at night and improve my health.

No, I'm referring to the undesirable type of fatigue, the one resulting from the stress I experience occasionally after having made blunders such as:
• drinking coffee in late-afternoon,
• overeating at dinnertime,

- getting caught in a sugar-eating binge,
- watching exciting, mostly stupid TV shows after dinner,
- permitting worries to invade my mind, etc.

You get the idea.

I'm "only human" and not immune to making such dumb mistakes. But it doesn't happen often any more. And when I stumble, I don't beat up on myself.

To stop counterproductive behavior in the bud and reconnect with my "better self," I resort to positive affirmations, deep breathing and other techniques.

Above all, I don't give up easily. If I fail, I simply try ... try ... and try again—until I succeed!

....

62. Persevere in establishing energizing habits

Chances are that most of us tried repeatedly to make lifestyle improvements, and had mixed results. We wanted to exercise more, relax more, eat less, cheer up, focus more on the essentials, plan more, check progress against plans, etc.

We start such initiatives with great hopes and enthusiasm—especially around the New Year and our birthdays, and we do, indeed, keep to our resolutions for a while.

> *But then we run into obstacles, get*
> *sidetracked, become discouraged*
> *and then give up ... again!*

If this ever happened to you: welcome to the club! Maybe you tried to change too quickly and fell flat on your face. Or maybe other, more pressing problems surfaced and took precedence.

> *Don't agonize over such failures.*
> *Don't let them diminish your self-*
> *esteem. Just dust yourself off and*
> *move on.*

Follow the best advice you can get, and take more time to make your improvements permanent.

But how much time?

In his hugely successful book, *Psycho-Cybernetics* (published in 1960), Maxwell Maltz stated that lifestyle changes can be made permanent in *21 days*. So according to him, it takes three weeks to establish new, lasting patterns of behavior.

Ever since, uncounted self-improvement gurus have mindlessly repeated this doctrine (although Maltz had never offered even just one shred of scientific evidence for it, but had based it merely on empirical observations).

As a result, it is now widely believed that it *does* indeed take 21 days to establish any worthwhile new habit.

His book is eminently worth studying. But this particular doctrine doesn't make sense to me at all. In my opinion, we need to *differentiate* in view of these facts:

- *The changes to be made differ widely.* Some detrimental practices can be dislodged easily with superior new habits from one moment to the next. Others (such as alcoholism) are more entrenched and may require months if not years of determined efforts to establish.

• *Individuals differ greatly as well.* Some of us can easily move ahead with giant strides. Others need to make changes far more slowly and gradually.

I may be able to get out of bed within minutes of waking up already on the day after having read that all it takes to make big changes is to shake off our negative psychological fixations. I would merely have to give up the erroneous belief that difficulties getting up in the morning are my "fate."

My belief system, physiology, etc., may indeed make it easy for me to jettison my time-wasting getting-up habit and to replace it with the practice of "just doing it" *at once.*

Similarly, I may also succeed in banishing French fries permanently from my dinner menus *from one day to the next* because I never liked them all that much.

But it may take me an entire week to get accustomed to chewing my food thoroughly (as postulated by Horace Fletcher), and it may take me *months* to overcome my practice of raiding the refrigerator before bedtime and senselessly gobbling up calorie-rich sleep-defying snacks and drinks.

Your performance may be far better than mine. Or worse.

> *Whatever time it may take to make*
> *changes is not nearly as important*
> *as persisting long enough for them*
> *to become permanent.*

The beneficial effects of superior new habits are worth our all-out efforts.

When you're stuck, and don't make any more headway, go back to the recommendations in this book. Read the sections on the life-changing benefits of moving your energy to much higher new levels (above, Part I, Sections B and C) to reinforce your motivation.

Then review the rest of the book again to re-discover the strategies you can choose from.

Use your judgment to adapt the recommendations to your personal circumstances and preferences where this appears to be to your advantage.

> *Experiment until you find the*
> *solution that's best for you.*

Move ahead, perhaps at a more deliberate pace. You may, for instance, want to focus exclusively on mastering *just one* particularly elusive improvement *for several weeks*.

> *Steady, controlled progress is better*
> *than trying to jump too high or too*
> *far, and ending up missing your goals.*

63. Progress the easy way—carried by a self-reinforcing upward spiral

Again, the main point is to persist. Don't give up until the good new habits are firmly entrenched.

Fortunately, the habits that you are working toward have their own, built-in reinforcements and rewards.

The more you put them to work for yourself, the more energetic and happy you'll become, and the better you will feel. And the better you feel, the more strength and courage you will gain, and the more motivated you'll become to make *even more and bolder improvements.*

Success in the areas of your life that you choose to focus on will become *progressively easier* to come by.

Success will build on success. You will become truly unstoppable!

So move ahead now! By initiating even minor improvements, you'll set a "virtuous cycle" in motion—an exciting self-reinforcing upward spiral that will keep motivating you to undertake ever-bolder new initiatives.

THANK YOU for having accompanied me all the way to the end of this book.

NOW PLEASE FOLLOW THROUGH WITH ACTION!

Take good care of yourself, and ENJOY THE EXHILARATING RIDE!

With best wishes for abundant energy, personal well-being, a steadfast can-do attitude and continuing success and satisfaction in all your endeavors:

Hugo Tschudin

P.S.

The following bonus section (K) gives you the essential information on the pros and cons of *sleep aids and medications.*

Please peruse it if you are currently using such products or might want to do so in the future.

Some of them are beneficial under the right circumstances. But even some of the best *herbal* products can have dangerous side effects, as you will see next.

K. The blessings and perils of sleep aids and medications

64. Be wary of sleep medications

Like food, money, work, exercise, relationships, sex and other important parts of our lives, *sleep medications can be good for us, or do us in.*

Sleep aids can mercifully end the terror of insomnia, and bring eagerly awaited and *perfectly legitimate relief* to individuals with difficulties falling and staying asleep.

But especially if used improperly, they can cause multiple *damaging side effects,* permanent physical and mental harm, life-threatening interactions with alcohol and other drugs, as well as life-long drug addiction.

> *Prescription- as well as non-prescription sleep medications should be used only as last resorts.*

Their use is justified only when strategies such as the ones described in this book don't work.

> *Moreover, medications should always be used only as long as necessary, and strictly within the guidelines of trustworthy medical practitioners or pharmacists.*

....

Hugo Tschudin's disclosure

I used prescription sleeping pills occasionally until a few years ago,
and I'm still keeping some leftovers in my night table for use
in an emergency ("just in case").

In the past—when I had a transatlantic consulting business
and conducted seminars in Europe on doing business in the
United States—I often turned to them for up to three nights
upon arrival in Europe, to overcome jet lag after my overnight
transatlantic flights.

In addition, I sometimes took sleeping pills at home for one or
two nights when I was upset and couldn't fall asleep without
them.

But in the *five years* prior to my writing the text you're
reading, I haven't felt any need to use sleeping pills any
longer because I usually practice what I preach.

I have disciplined myself to keep worries and frustrations
under control and to calm myself down—making liberal use
of affirmations and relaxation techniques—by the time I'm
ready for bed.

....

65. What you should know about prescription sleep medications

Prescription sleeping pills ("hypnotics") are the *most effective*
remedies for insomnia but also carry the *highest risks*.

Particularly hazardous are sleeping pills containing *benzo-diapines,* such as Restoril and Halcion. Fortunately, they are rarely used today; medical practitioners prescribe them only when there's a pressing need for them.

Today's "bestsellers" are the more recent *benzodiapine-free medications.* But even these (such as Ambien, Sonata, and Lunesta) should be used with great restraint for a variety of reasons:

* They *suppress rapid-eye-movement (REM) sleep,* thus preventing users from getting totally restorative sleep.
* They sometimes *cause undesirable behaviors* such as falls (when sleepers get up at night), sleep-walking, sleep-eating and even sleep-driving.
* They carry risks such as *morning hangovers* and *daytime sleepiness* (which may cause traffic, workplace and other *accidents,* and may also *impair performance* on and off the job, cause *memory loss,* etc.).
* They *don't solve the underlying causes* of insomnia. Rather, they help to cover them up and perpetuate them.
* They may lead to *psychological dependency,* life-long *addiction* and even *chronic insomnia (!).*
* They are extremely *dangerous* for individuals who are also *drinking alcohol* or using other sedating drugs.

> *Without case-specific approval by a reputable medical practitioner, prescription sleep medications should be used only for coping with temporary problems (such as upsetting short-term stress, or jet lag).*

They should never be used for more than a week.

66. Don't assume that non-prescription sleep medications are harmless

Because the so-called over-the-counter (OTC) medications are available without doctors' prescriptions, they are generally—but *wrongly—believed to be innocuous.*

They usually contain *antihistamines such as diphenhydramine hydrochloride.*

These ingredients are used mainly to suppress symptoms of colds and allergies. But because they *induce drowsiness,* they are also marketed as sleep aids. They do, indeed, make it somewhat easier to fall asleep.

Regrettably, they induce *shallow rather than deep sleep.*

Worse still, *they share many of the side effects of prescription sleeping pills,* such as dangerous drug interactions, morning hangovers, daytime sleepiness and its attendant accident and other risks.

> *As mentioned on their labels, they should be avoided by persons with bronchitis, breathing problems and glaucoma as well as by women who are pregnant or nursing.*

67. What you should know about herbal sleep aids

The most popular herbal sleep aids are VALERIAN, CHA-MOMILE, PASSIONFLOWER and KAVA KAVA. Available without prescriptions, they are widely reputed to have calming effects and to promote falling and remaining asleep.

But some observers believe them to have mostly—or only—*placebo effects*. This is, of course, hardly objectionable to persons for whom they are effective.

Because herbal sleep aids can't be patented, the business community is rarely interested in researching their properties.

> *Their long-term effects and possible interaction with certain other medications and medical conditions are largely unknown.*

So it would be wrong to assume that they are totally safe. They should be used in moderation and cautiously.

(1) VALERIAN, the most popular herbal sleep supplement, is available in the form of drops, capsules and soft gels made from the plant's roots.

Valerian is reputed to *increase the release of serotonin,* a relaxing, "feel-good" neurotransmitter. It does not cause any hangovers, nor does it reduce the patient's alertness.

Valerian is, however, not to be used by children and adolescents with attention-deficit hyperactivity disorder (ADHD).

According to a recent study of the Norwegian Knowledge Center for Health Services, Valerian has little or no effect on sleep. But some survey participants staunchly vouched for its effectiveness.

(2) CHAMOMILE has, for centuries, enjoyed the reputation of "calming one's soul." It's used as an infusion (tea) made from the dried yellow flower heads of the chamomile plant, and available also in the form of drops.

Its effective agents (particularly the *flavonoid apigenin*) make it not only a *gentle sleep aid*, but also *relieve stomach irritations and gas,* and fight ulcers and inflammations.

Chamomile has no serious side effects (but is allergenic for the rare individuals who are allergic to daisies).

> *Chamomile should, however, be avoided by patients taking blood thinners and by pregnant women.*

(3) PASSIONFLOWER is another herbal product that *calms the central nervous system and promotes sleep.* It's available in tea and drop form.

> *Passionflower should not be taken with sedatives such as anti-histamines, anti-anxiety products or other sleep remedies.*

<u>(4) KAVA KAVA.</u> This herbal supplement may be more effective than the previous three. There's some "serious" scientific evidence of its efficacy.

Available without prescription in health food and other stores (as teas, drops and capsules made with extracts of powdered roots), its *effects resemble the ones of alcohol, marijuana and Valium* to some degree, but without the hangover effect of—for instance—alcoholic nightcaps.

> *In fact, kava kava makes sleepers*
> *wake up highly energized because*
> *of its sleep-deepening effect.*

WARNING: Before rushing to a health-food store to buy Kava Kava, please consider the *downside*. Consumption in large quantities may result in *liver damage*. Not surprisingly, packages of kava products contain some safety warnings.

68. What you should know about the increasingly popular non-herbal sleep supplement melatonin

Particularly noteworthy among *non-herbal* insomnia supplements is melatonin.

Melatonin is *a "sleep hormone"* secreted by the brain's pineal gland when our surroundings turn dark. The absence of light induces drowsiness and sleep in this process *naturally*.

We can speed up this occurrence by consuming man-made melatonin. Synthesized by industry, this hormone is widely available at low cost as a prescription-free food supplement in the United States, but sold exclusively by prescription in many other countries (including Canada and most of Western Europe).

In the USA, melatonin is most often used in the form of tablets of 3 or 5 milligram. Recent research showed that even a mere one-third to one-tenth (!) of this dosage can be as effective as entire tablets.

Some researchers speculate that melatonin may be particularly beneficial for sleep-deprived *older adults* because their pineal glands may have become less productive.

In addition to its use as a sleep aid (for overcoming jet lag and the consequences of shift work, etc.), melatonin can assist in the fight against a multitude of illnesses.

WARNING: Before buying melatonin from a health food or other store or by mail order, please consider this:

- Some aspects of the use and effects of melatonin are still unknown or controversial.

- As a powerful hormone, melatonin *can* be dangerous. There are a few drug-interaction dangers and other good reasons for the restrictions placed on its sale in many advanced foreign countries.

> *Melatonin should not be used by children, pregnant women and women trying to get pregnant as well as by persons with autoimmune diseases, lymphoma and certain other types of cancer, depression*

> *and mental illnesses, severe aller-*
> *gies, etc.*

Because of its effectiveness as a sleep aid, its power to fight certain illnesses, and because of its *high antioxidant content*, melatonin appears to be gaining favor also in the traditional medical community.

> *Please observe the warnings*
> *found on the labels of melato-*
> *inn bottles. Better still, consult*
> *a medical practitioner before*
> *using this hormone.*

....

Hugo Tschudin's disclosure

In the past, *I often used 3-milligram melatonin tablets.*

After having read that much smaller quantities can have the same sleep-inducing effect, I cut my usage down to one-half, then one fourth and even less of a tablet. To my surprise, the changes indeed didn't make any difference.

Intrigued by this experiment, I took it to the next level: I quit taking melatonin altogether.

This, again, did not alter the outcome. I had no trouble falling asleep. So I began wondering if melatonin had only a placebo effect on sleeplessness.

Because an increasing number of conventional and holistic healthcare providers have given higher overall marks to melatonin (particularly emphasizing its high antioxidant power), *I started using melatonin again.*

I'm taking 1.5 milligram (one-half of the most common tablet size) upon going to bed, and the same quantity upon going back to bed after bathroom breaks.

Because individuals' needs differ, *I encourage you again to experiment*—with the approval of a knowledgeable medical practitioner, of course.

....

69. What you should know about tryptophan

Tryptophan is a *precursor of* the body's production of the "feel-good hormone" *serotonin*, and serotonin can, in turn, be converted into the "sleep hormone" melatonin.

> *Like melatonin, tryptophan has*
> *a relaxing effect and promotes*
> *healthy sleep.*

Lack of tryptophan (and serotonin) can lead to *insomnia*, fatigue, depression, anxiety, low concentration and low self-esteem.

Tryptophan is an *essential* amino acid, which means that we must obtain it from our diet (or a supplement).

Excellent natural sources of tryptophan include:
• soybeans (the consumption of which might lead to health problems in men),
• milk, cheese and other dairy products,

• turkey, chicken and other types of meat, and fish, and
• sunflower and other seeds.

Incidentally, the tryptophan in turkey is vastly overestimated. Turkey does not contain significantly more tryptophan than other types of meat, or fish. In addition, the tryptophan in a turkey meal is unlikely to stimulate the production of serotonin significantly for a *second* reason: because it must compete with too many other amino acids.

Very little of the turkey's tryptophan reaches the brain to help produce serotonin.

> *Fatigue and drowsiness in the wake of a Thanksgiving or Christmas feast are caused mostly by what is consumed alongside of the turkey — especially carbohydrates and alcohol — rather than by the turkey's tryptophan.*

In the United States, tryptophan is available without prescription as a *food supplement*, for instance in the form of capsules containing 500 mg.

L-tryptophan, the L-version of this amino acid, is reported to be its most effective form.

> *Tryptophan supplements should not be taken together with protein (such as turkey!) because they interfere with protein absorption (!).*

....

Hugo Tschudin's Personal Note

I don't use any tryptophan preparations because *melatonin* is highly effective as a sleep aid, has antioxidant properties, and is available widely at low cost in the United States.

....

RESOURCES THAT WILL KEEP YOU "IN THE FLOW"

There's no need to put up with frequent fatigue ... nor the "blahs" ... nor a hum-drum life.

The following know-how sources are valuable guides to, and re-minders of, a much more energetic, dynamic, productive and happy "New You."

(1) EnergizingLife Newsletter (f.r.e.e.)

Published monthly via the Internet, this newsletter:

• *Presents energizing strategies, actionable tips and inspiring success stories.*

• *Helps readers to increase their energy for greater success and satisfaction.*

• *Reminds and motivates readers, and makes it easy for them to maintain powerful forward momentum.*

VISIT <u>EnergizingLife.com</u> for this f.r.e.e. service.

Subscribing and unsubscribing take mere seconds, and your information will never be shared with others.

(2) Wake Up to Abundant Energy: 113 Ways to "Rise and Shine" (DOWNLOADS, US $1.99)

This is a complete, time-saving ACTION PROGRAM, condensed into 20 information-packed pages with OVER 100 ACTIONABLE TIPS.

It describes:

• *10 routines making getting out of bed easy and even fun,*

• *10 vigor-boosting bedroom arrangements,*

• *6 ways to avoid sleep interruptions, or to take them in stride,*

• *10 strategies to end the terror of alarm clocks (including three to get rid of them entirely).*

• *Directions for becoming MORE energetic with LESS sleep (of special interest to go-getters who dislike sleeping their lives away!).*

VISIT EnergizingLife.com to download this empowering program for only US $1.99.

(3) Wake Up to Abundant Energy: 113 Ways to "Rise and Shine' (PRINTED booklets)

This is the same as the "downloads"described above but is available *on a limited basis* in the form of elegant, top-quality

PRINTED booklets with glossy four-color front and back covers.

• *Convenient to carry in vest pockets and hand bags.*

• *Suitable for mailing in regular long (No.10) envelopes.*

• *Life-changing, and likely to be kept for years to come.*

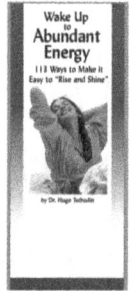

Single copies are available ONLY at Hugo Tschudin's semi-nars and lectures, for US $3.00.

(4) Wake up to Abundant Energy: 113 Ways to "Rise and Shine" (LICENSES to print booklets)

Have booklets produced under license (with your logo and other imprints if desired).

• *DISTRIBUTE THEM TO EMPLOYEES to: create goodwill ... help them to get up easily (even on Mondays!) ... reduce late arrivals and absenteeism ... help employees to stay alert, fight fatigue and keep up with demanding work.*

• *USE BOOKLETS AS INCENTIVES for: requesting literature, offers, etc. ... visiting stores, trade show booths, doctors' offices, etc. ... ordering products, subscribing, joining organizations, etc.*

• *KEEP BOOKLETS HANDY AS SMALL GIFTS for: favors, orders, payments, testimonials, etc.*

ADDITIONAL INFORMATION: htschudin@tschudin.com.